International Co-operation in Health

OXFORD
UNIVERSITY PRESS

Great Clarendon Street, Oxford OX2 6DP

Oxford University Press is a department of the University of Oxford.
It furthers the University's objective of excellence in research, scholarship,
and education by publishing worldwide in

Oxford New York

Athens Auckland Bangkok Bogotá Buenos Aires Cape Town
Chennai Dar es Salaam Delhi Florence Hong Kong Istanbul Karachi
Kolkata Kuala Lumpur Madrid Melbourne Mexico City Mumbai Nairobi
Paris São Paulo Shanghai Singapore Taipei Tokyo Toronto Warsaw

with associated companies in Berlin Ibadan

Oxford is a registered trade mark of Oxford University Press
in the UK and in certain other countries

Published in the United States
by Oxford University Press Inc., New York

British Library Cataloguing in Publication Data

Data available

Library of Congress Cataloguing in Publication Data

ISBN 0-19-263198-5

10 9 8 7 6 5 4 3 2 1

Typeset by EXPO Holdings, Malaysia
Printed in Great Britain
on acid-free paper by Biddles Ltd, Guildford & King's Lynn

International Co-operation in Health

Edited by

Martin McKee
Professor of European Public Health, London School of Hygiene and Tropical Medicine

Paul Garner
Professor of International Health, Liverpool School of Tropical Medicine

Robin Stott
Consultant Physician, Lewisham University Hospital and Chairman MEDACT, London

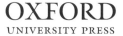

OXFORD
UNIVERSITY PRESS

Preface

How is the health of the public affected by globalization? How can health professionals engage in the changes happening in the world around them? These questions arose in discussions between the editors, in mid–1999, about the challenges to population health that were emerging as a consequence of globalization.

Working out what globalization means to people is the first step, so that people have a common understanding. We were equally concerned about the capacity of the global public health community to respond. We each had considerable experience working with international agencies and we had significant reservations about their ability to develop, co-ordinate and implement effective policies. On the other hand, we knew that this situation was changing. In particular, under new leadership, the World Health Organization was placing a much higher priority on some of the key issues. We wanted to know what the international agencies were doing and what challenges they faced.

Non-governmental agencies have a role in the process, and one of the editorial team is a member of MEDACT, a non-governmental organization devoted to giving health professionals a voice in some of the major issues facing the world today. This perspective recognizes the role of governments and international agencies but also stresses that everyone, and especially health professionals, can play a part.

It's a rapidly changing field, and not possible to be comprehensive in our coverage. We therefore focused on some of the issues facing the health of the population of the world at the beginning of the twenty-first century. There are other issues boiling up, including trade in illicit drugs, the emerging international framework for intellectual property rights, debt, and debt relief, and many more others. We have, however, tried to include some of what we believe are the major issues facing the global health community today. We have sought to set out the scale of the challenges we face, the opportunities that exist, the responses that are being developed and, most importantly, what we can do as individuals.

There are many people without whom this book would not have been possible. Kelley Lee and Gill Walt have been helpful at all times; the authors of our chapters have responded with considerable tolerance to our continuing demands to meet deadlines and to revise their contributions. Caroline White was an enormous help in preparing and formatting the references. Helen Liepman, at Oxford University Press, provided unstinting support and almost saint-like tolerance as we missed deadlines. Finally, we must thank our families for their continuing support.

Contents

List of Contributors

Orvill Adams
Director, Department of Organization of
Health Services Delivery
World Health Organization
20 Avenue Appia
1211 Geneva
Switzerland

Douglas W. Bettcher
Coordinator, Framework Convention on
Tobacco Control Team
Tobacco Free Initiative
World Health Organization
20 Avenue Appia
1211 Geneva
Switzerland

Oona Campbell
Senior Lecturer
Department of Infectious and Tropical
Diseases
London School of Hygiene and Tropical
Medicine
Keppel Street
London WC1E 7HT
UK

Julio Frenk
Minister of Health
Secretaria de Salud
Lieja 7
06696 Mexico, D.F.
Mexico

Douglas Holdstock
Retired consultant physician
MEDACT
601 Holloway Rd
London
N19 4DJ
UK

Kelley Lee
Senior Lecturer in Global Health Policy
London School of Hygiene and Tropical
Medicine
Keppel Street
London WC1E 7HT
UK

Louisiana Lush
Lecturer
Centre for Population Studies
London School of Hygiene and Tropical
Medicine
50 Bedford Square
London WC1B 3DP
UK

Emmanuela E. Gakidou
Health Economist
Evidence and Information for Policy
Cluster
World Health Organization
20 Avenue Appia
1211 Geneva
Switzerland

Paul Garner
Professor of International Health
Liverpool School of Tropical Medicine
Liverpool
L17 7BD
UK

Octavio Gómez-Dantés,
Director of Evaluation
Secretaria de Salud
Lieja 7
06696 Mexico, D.F.
Mexico

Tim Lang
Professor of Food Policy
Centre for Food Policy
Thames Valley University
St Mary's Road, Ealing
London W5 5RF
UK

Martin McKee
Professor of European Public Health
London School of Hygiene and
Tropical Medicine
Keppel Street
London WC1E 7HT
UK

Tony McMichael
Professor of Epidemiology
Department of Epidemiology and
Population Health
London School of Hygiene and Tropical
Medicine
Keppel Street
London WC1E 7HT
UK

Harry Minas
Director, Centre for International
Mental Health
Director, Victorian Transcultural
Psychiatry Unit
University of Melbourne
St. Vincent's Hospital
Nicholson Street
Fitzroy, Victoria 3065
Australia

Robin Stott
Consultant Physician
MEDACT
601 Holloway Rd
London
N19 4DJ
UK

Chitra Subramaniam,
Coordinator, External Relations
Tobacco Free Initiative
World Health Organization,
20 Avenue Appia
1211 Geneva
Switzerland

Allyn L. Taylor
Legal adviser
Tobacco Free Initiative
World Health Organization,
20 Avenue Appia
1211 Geneva
Switzerland

Julius Weinberg
Pro Vice-chancellor (Research)
City University
Northampton Square
London EC1 0HV
UK

Heather Wipfli
Technical officer
Tobacco Free Initiative
World Health Organization,
20 Avenue Appia
1211 Geneva
Switzerland

Alistair Woodward
Professor of Public Health
Wellington School of Medicine
Wellington
New Zealand

Chapter 1

Introduction

Martin McKee, Robin Stott, and Paul Garner

A historical perspective

As the twenty-first century dawns, there is a rapidly increasing public awareness of the imbalance between the global reach of factors that affect human health and the inadequate structures in place to address them. Those suffering as a result of forest fires in Montana, flooded rivers in England, and drought in Kenya are aware that their climate is changing, almost certainly because of the activities of man, but feel powerless to respond. Health professionals seeking to curb the spread of tobacco through the developing world struggle against the enormous resources of trans-national companies that ignore bans on advertising and blanket cities with their logos. Local communities discover that their local hospital has been taken over by a trans-national health care corporation that seeks to expand its profits by market segmentation, in effect excluding them from care.

But it is easy to overlook how global factors have always exerted an influence on human health. The earliest examples arose from changes in the natural environment. Some are obvious, even if the precise effects on human health remain shrouded in uncertainty, such as the last ice age (Young 1983). Others are less obvious but are being identified by an increasing number of imaginative analyses by historians that draw on a wide range of sources to connect events that took place in different parts of the world. Thus, historians have long been aware of a major change in the climate of Europe in the sixth century AD that coincided with widespread migration, including the Anglo-Saxon invasion of England, which were facilitated by the unusually high river levels at the time, thus enabling the invaders to penetrate much further inland than would have previously been possible (Davies 1999). Keys has linked these events with a volcanic eruption off the coast of Java in AD 535, that led to global atmospheric cooling (Keys 1999). He shows how this, in turn, caused failure of harvests and, in Eurasia, migration of populations and spread of plague, and the emergence of many of the national groupings that now make up western Europe (Box 1.1). Several centuries later, the little ice age which stretched from the fourteenth to the seventeenth century had important consequences for many populations, such as the elimination through famine and disease, of the long established Viking settlements in Greenland (Gribbin and Gribbin 1990; McMichael 2001). Finally, a recent analysis of famines and droughts in Africa and Asia in the 1870s, catalogued in some detail by the journalists following the former US President Ulysses Grant who was on a world tour at the time, has shown how the consequences of global climatic events, in this case El Niño, were exacerbated by the recent advent of a global market that had undermined the indigenous support mechanisms that had coped successfully with a similar event a century earlier (Davis 2001). These events had major and lasting implications for the economic relationship between Africa and Asia on the one hand and Europe and North America on the other.

Box 1.1: **Catastrophe – the impact of climate change on human history**

In AD 535 and 536 the world experienced a momentous series of climatic events. The sun became dim for up to 18 months. From China, to Europe, to the Americas, crops failed and famine ensued. The worst floods and droughts in living memory were described everywhere that written records existed. Elsewhere, archaeological evidence shows how, for several years, tree growth virtually ceased. Plague spread out of southern China and ultimately all the way across Europe.

David Keys has assembled a large body of evidence showing that these changes led to the collapse of empires in Europe and America, including the western Roman Empire and the Mexican Empire of Teotihucan. These paved the way for the emergence of new political forces, such as the Frankish Empire, the Mayans, the Ottomans, and a unified China, thus creating the political and economic groupings that form the basis of the modern world. He shows how these climatic events can be linked to the eruption of a volcano in the sea off Java, close to the island of Krakatoa which itself exploded in AD 1883. This eruption may be the first example in recorded history of how global climate change can change the course of world events.

From the thirteenth century onwards, human activity began to impact globally on health. McNeill shows how two events, the opening of the Straits of Gibraltar to Christian shipping by the Genoese in 1291 and the development of trade routes across the Eurasian steppe by the Mongols created the conditions by which plague could spread throughout Europe after 1346 (McNeil 1976).

The European conquest of the Americas offered many opportunities for the spread of disease as two populations that had developed in isolation from each other, exposed to, and thus acquiring immunity to different infectious diseases, came into contact with one another. It seems likely that the appearance of syphilis in Europe, in 1493, arose from the participation in the siege of Naples of Spanish sailors, who had acquired the disease on their trip with Columbus, with the inevitable orgy of rape and pillage and who had acquired the disease on the trip (Porter 1997). The consequences of Columbus's journey for the Native American population were, however vastly greater. Conditions in Eurasia had favoured the development of agriculture and domestication of animals, from which Europeans acquired a wide range of initially zoonotic infections, such as measles. These were unknown in the Americas. A single case of smallpox that reached Mexico in 1520 is estimated to have contributed directly to the decline of about 90 per cent in the Native American population over the following century (Diamond 1997).

As international trade developed, the association with health slowly became apparent. One aspect was the opportunity provided by trading vessels to spread infectious diseases (Chapter 4), leading first to the system of quarantine and later to international health regulations. Another was trade in goods that, while profitable for those transporting and selling the goods, had adverse consequences for health. An early example was opium, which was so lucrative that the UK prepared to go to war with China in 1840 and again in 1857 for the right to export it freely. In the twentieth century western governments disengaged from the international trade in narcotics (except for occasional ventures linked to covert military operations) and have actively sought to suppress it. Paradoxically, some countries, especially those that host head offices of trans-national tobacco corporations, have continued to support the expansion of global trade in another addictive drug, nicotine, which has much greater consequences for the global burden of disease.

Many of the events mentioned so far have been associated, in one way or another, with conflict, whether as cause or effect. Pressure on natural resources, whether due to overgrazing of land or climate change, has been a frequent cause of war, most recently in Rwanda (Shawcross 2000). The global trade in minerals, especially diamonds, has created a malign network of gem and arms traders, creating new trade routes between diamond-bearing countries such as Sierra Leone, arms exporters such as Bulgaria and Ukraine and diamond processors such as Belgium. At last, the international diamond trade has recognized its role in the process by which tens of thousands of African children have had their limbs severed in the cause of international trade. Unfortunately, wars such as that in the Democratic Republic of the Congo continue to be fuelled by the struggle to control mineral resources.

The victims of wars in Africa are only some of the many people who find themselves caught up in wars whose origins, if they were understood at all, must have seemed very remote. Europe too has fallen victim to the consequences of events elsewhere, especially in central Asia. Examples include the westward movement of the Huns in the sixth century, the Mongol raids of the thirteenth century and the fall of Constantinople in 1453.

Thus, an important lesson from history is how local events can have global repercussions that are difficult to predict. In 1914, few Americans, Canadians, or South Africans could have imagined, even if they were aware at the time that the event had happened, that the assassination of an Austrian archduke in Sarajevo would lead, within four years, to many thousands of their compatriots dying on the fields of Flanders.

It would, however, be wrong to present global factors as entirely negative. Movements of people and goods have had hugely beneficial effects on human health. The spread of crops and livestock has vastly improved nutrition and supported the growth of populations everywhere. The global diffusion of knowledge, whether about improved ways of organizing one's business, manufacturing a better product or delivering health care, has made a huge contribution to the improvement of the human condition. Again, this is a process with a long history. The Abbasids, in Baghdad, took up and translated the ancient Greek texts on medicine, so enabling them to be reintroduced into western Europe by Arabic scholars in Salerno and Toledo several centuries after they had been forgotten in Europe. This provided the foundation for modern scientific medicine.

The spread of ideas was however, slow, complex and subject to local interpretation. Thus, the basic ideas about the causation of disease, developed by the Greeks and later by the Arabs, were taken across the Sahara by traders, to reappear in a modified form among the beliefs of the descendants of slaves transported to the Caribbean (Leigh-Fermor 1984). By the end of the twentieth century, this process had been transformed by the Internet, creating the concept of the global electronic village.

Emerging concerns

So if human health has always been subject to global influences, why does there seem to be more concern about it now? Why has the term 'globalization' entered popular usage and what does it actually mean? And why did thousands of people converge on Seattle at the end of 1999 to protest about 'world trade'?

Although this book is not primarily about the process of 'globalization' the concept is central to it. For this reason, we begin with an exploration of its meaning and implications.

Kelley Lee (Chapter 2) identifies three dimensions of globalization. The first relates to how we understand the physical space we inhabit. The world is increasingly seen as a global village (McLuhan and Powers 1989). Europeans and Americans whose grandparents might never have moved from their own village now take holidays on the opposite side of the world. They may even lift their telephone in London to make their reservation with a British airline but be connected with someone working in a call centre in New Delhi. Some countries that are geographically isolated and with few natural resources have developed innovative ways to exploit these possibilities (Box 1.2).

Box 1.2: Tuvalu – exploiting the global economy

Tuvalu, an archipelago in the South Pacific, that was known as the Ellice Islands during the colonial period, offers an example of how small states can exploit the emerging global economy (Stanley, 2000). Tuvalu consists of nine low-lying atolls, with a total land area of only 25 square kilometres. It exports only small quantities of locally manufactured clothing, some fish and copra, and imports almost all its food and manufactured goods. Despite these circumstances, Tuvalu has no foreign debt. It has achieved this position by taking full advantage of a diverse set of international activities. One source of revenue is the Tuvalu Trust Fund, established with initial contributions from the UK, Australia and New Zealand. The fund is invested in the global capital market, doubling in value between 1987 and 1998. A second source is income from licence fees from American, Korean, and Taiwanese boats fishing for tuna within Tuvalu's exclusive economic zone, established under the provisions of the 1982 UN treaty on the Law of the Sea. A third source is the

Box 1.2: **Tuvalu – exploiting the global economy** (continued)

income arising from the sale of telephone sex lines to operators using the excess capacity on the Tuvalu telephone exchange, established by the Australian government's aid programme as a means of improving inter-island communication. Tuvalu avoids some of the potential problems that might arise from this arrangement by preventing access to the services from Tuvalu and ensuring that the operators are based elsewhere, mostly in Australia. Since 1998, Tuvalu has taken advantage of its Internet suffix,. tv, to market domain names at US$1000 each, although this venture has been less successful than the others. Finally, the Tuvalu government has also engaged in widespread sales of passports, primarily to Hong Kong Chinese.

The second relates to the pace with which we interact with the rest of the world. Long-range aeroplanes fly non-stop from London to Singapore, at prices that have continually fallen in real terms. Electronic mail provides a low-cost means to work in teams across continents. A global financial market has been created with London, New York and Tokyo providing 24-hour opportunities to buy and sell.

The third relates to the spread of global culture, ideas, and beliefs. Teenagers in Atlanta, Johannesburg, Berlin and Tokyo will be equally familiar with the symbols of McDonald's and Coca-Cola and will watch the same Hollywood films. On the 31 December 1999 people all over the world joined together in an extravaganza of fireworks and celebrations, to celebrate the birth of a new millennium. But many will also be aware of the key issues in debates about the environment, human rights, or debt relief.

Several specific manifestations of these dimensions are of particular importance for health. First is the way in which the changing nature of the world, and its implications for health, is increasingly being manifest in ways that are apparent to the public. Television cameras bring wars across the world into people's living rooms. Increases in insurance bills are attributed to the consequences of a more unpredictable climate, itself a manifestation of global warming. Outbreaks of infectious disease are linked to failures in food processing plants in another part of the world.

The second is the extent to which national governments are increasingly seen as powerless in the face of global influences. Concern has been greatest about the growing power of trans-national corporations, now underpinned by the authority of the World Trade Organization (WTO). Thus, attempts by European governments to ban the import of hormone-treated beef, reflecting widely held concerns among their populations about its safety, were found to be unlawful. Of potentially greater concern is the scope for global processes to undermine established rights of employees and welfare systems, either indirectly by shifting production to poorer countries with less well-developed social protection mechanisms or more directly by inclusion of services in future world trade rounds (Rodrik 1997). Another concern is the way in which people across the world suddenly discover that the intellectual property rights to the crops they have grown for generations or the plants they have used as medicines have been appropriated by biotechnology companies in the west.

The third is a breakdown of trust in authority (McKee and Lang 1996). In the past many people would have been willing to accept reassurances of 'experts'. This is no longer so following a series of events, such as the BSE affair in the UK (McKee *et al.* 1996) or scandals with contaminated blood in France and Germany. More recently, attempts by large agro-chemical companies to market products based on genetic modification have confronted profound public suspicion in many countries, to such an extent that involvement with such products is seen by many retailers as a substantial liability. Scientific 'experts' are now often perceived to be either out of touch with the concerns of the public or to be under the influence of corporate interests. Distrust in politicians has also increased, fuelled by media exposure of scandals such as the apparent link between a large political donation and the British government's decision to promote the postponement of a Europe-wide ban on tobacco sponsorship.

Fourth, the consequences of international factors are often insidious, with the chain of causation convoluted and obscure. A conventional, uni-disciplinary model of research, coupled with inadequate data and a lack of lateral thinking, has often failed to unravel these links.

Traditional epidemiological methods, such as cohort and case-control studies, have failed to rise to the challenge of defining exposure to such factors as climate change or trade policies. Alternative approaches, triangulating evidence from multiple sources and using ecological designs, have too often been dismissed as unscientific by an establishment that has failed to grasp the importance of some of the big challenges facing humanity. This is now changing, as researchers adopt innovative methods and use new data sets, an example being the work that has quantified the diverse health effects of the El Niño phenomenon in the southern Pacific Ocean (Bouma *et al.* 1997). Similarly, work to map patterns of antibiotic resistance among bacteria has shown the importance of failure by some countries to control prescribing effectively, coupled with a larger volume of international travel. Such approaches are making the previously invisible effects of far-off events visible.

The history of international action on health

Until relatively recently, two features have characterized discussions on governance in the field of international health. First, these discussions have remained largely concerned with the tension between the free movement of goods and people and the control of epidemic disease. Second, they have been conducted primarily between states.

As noted earlier, the relative lack of geographical barriers in the Eurasian land mass did much to foster international trade and increased prosperity but this brought in its wake the threat of infectious disease, especially plague. For several centuries the policy of quarantine, initially introduced by the Venetians but subsequently adopted throughout western Europe, was an effective means of control, but by the middle of the nineteenth century, it confronted two major challenges. The first was the increasing volume and, especially, the speed of trade due to the introduction of the railway and the steamship. Delays due to quarantine were increasingly costly and unacceptable. The second was the appearance in Europe of cholera, a disease that the existing arrangements seemed unable to control (Fidler 1999).

With the twin aims of protecting Europe from cholera while facilitating international trade, the first International Sanitary Conference convened in Paris in 1851, attended by government representatives of twelve countries. The subsequent sequence of events provided the first of many examples of the difficulties in agreeing action on international health. Although delegates supported the proposal that cholera be subject to quarantine regulations, their governments were unable to ratify this decision. It was not until many International Sanitary Conferences later that governments, meeting in Venice in 1892, were able to reach a limited agreement to impose quarantine on ships that actually had cases of cholera on board. The subsequent International Sanitary Conferences did lead to the establishment of a permanent International Committee on Epidemics, in 1874, and the adoption of the International Sanitary Convention (ISC). Successive conferences paved the way for the present mechanisms for international control of infectious disease, such as the establishment of an International Surveillance System covering certain communicable diseases. It was, however, only in 1903 that the ISC reached agreement that states would 'immediately notify the other governments of the first appearance in its territory of authentic cases of plague or cholera' (Fidler 1999).

In 1907, European governments established a new body, the Office International d'Hygiène Publique (OIHP), in Paris, with the task of collecting and disseminating information on infectious diseases, broadening its interests progressively from the traditional concerns of the west, plague, cholera, and yellow fever, to encompass diseases such as malaria, tuberculosis, and typhoid (Porter 1997). After the First World War, however, the League of Nations was established and with it a Health Organization. The obvious course would have been to merge the League's Health Organization with the OIHP and with the recently established Pan-American Sanitary Bureau and the older Maritime and Quarantine Sanitary Council in Alexandria. However the USA, which was now a member of the OIHP but not of the League of Nations, vetoed the move.

The list of international bodies created after the Second World War, within the framework of the United Nations (UN), included the World Health Organization (WHO). The WHO was given the role of directing and co-ordinating action on international health but with the proviso that it could only act in a country with the approval of its government (Goodman 1971). For much of the post-war period the leading role of the WHO in international health was unquestioned and it had many major successes, most notably the eradication of smallpox.

More recently, however, the international arena has become much more crowded. Some of the new entrants are also international organizations, such as the World Bank, especially after the publication of its landmark 1993 World Development Report, *Investing in health* (World Bank 1993). Although criticized because of the health consequences of its structural adjustment policies, it has also made major contributions such as its participation in the measurement of the global burden of disease (Murray and Lopez 1996) and in extending the understanding of the economics of tobacco consumption (Jha and Chaloupka 1999). Other UN agencies have also become more influential in international health, including the United Nations Children's Fund (UNICEF), the United Nations Development Programme (UNDP) and the United Nations Population Fund (UNPF).

But there are also other new players (Koivusalo and Ollial 1997). Some, such as the WTO, may not have been thought of initially as participating in the development of international health policy but are now seen as important players with regard to many of the tradable determinants of health. For others, such as the Organization for Economic Co-operation and Development (OECD) and the regional development banks, health may be a side issue but their overall importance on the international scene makes them significant players.

So far, however, this analysis has been limited to a traditional model of international relations, based on states and intergovernmental organizations. Such an analysis is, however, becoming rapidly obsolete. States are extremely heterogeneous and some of the new non-governmental players are vastly more influential than, say, a micro-state in the Caribbean or Pacific Ocean, with a population of a few thousand. Indeed, the 50 largest trans-national corporations have sales revenues greater than 131 members of the UN. The private sector is a major player and it is increasingly able to circumvent attempts by states to regulate it, whether by exploiting extra-territoriality, manipulating transfer prices between subsidiaries in different countries to avoid taxes, or through direct or indirect pressure on governments. Interestingly, when the issue relates to something important, such as money, but not health, it seems that governments can take effective concerted action, as in the Basle Committee that lays down standards for the viability of commercial banks. Such examples are, however, rare.

Another new entrant is the non-governmental organization (NGO). Judged by membership, the largest of these are also somewhat larger than many countries. They can also be more influential. Some large international bodies are actually global NGOs, often working closely with the intergovernmental agencies. An example is the International Air Transport Association (IATA), formed by the world's airlines, which collaborates closely with the International Civil Aviation Organization (ICAO), a UN specialized agency. In other situations, organizations such as the International Committee of the Red Cross (ICRC), NGOs, and governments participate as equals. Yet other NGOs may have less formal links with governments but, by virtue of their wide networks and specialized expertise, they make extremely effective inputs to policy. Examples include the Rockefeller and Ford Foundations, Oxfam, and the Open Society Institute. Finally, the past decade has seen a rapid growth in grass roots direct action organizations (Klein 1999). An early example was BUGA UP, an Australian group that used spray paint to distort tobacco advertisements. More recent ones include Reclaim the Streets, who blockade roads in protest about a lack of effective transport policies and the Biotic Baking Brigade, who seek to deflate the leaders of trans-national corporations by throwing cream pies at them.

But even this list is incomplete. In some areas of health policy another type of organization is active. International criminal groups must be taken into account in the debate about how to address the use of narcotics. Crime is also increasingly recognized as a brake on social and economic development, with implications for health, in particular because of the way that it inhibits the growth of small and medium enterprises and by its direct impact on mental health.

Thus, an analysis of the global policy environment that is limited to nation states and international agencies is incomplete. It is essential to take into account the diverse range of other contributors. This has major implications for the process of policy making. At last, the vision of a 'global open society' seems realizable (Soros 1998), subject to scrutiny by the media, by civic society, and ultimately by the public.

Who is this book for?

This book is primarily about international collaboration to promote the health of the world's population. Such collaboration can be at many levels, ranging from international agencies to individuals. It aims to highlight how international collaboration can and does help to tackle current and emerging public health problems.

It is not, however, a map of the existing institutional responses to global health challenges. This has already been covered very well by others (Koivusalo and Ollial 1997). Instead, this book is predicated on the belief that concerted international action by health professionals is one means of bringing about change. Although, to some, the idea that individuals can make a difference in the face of enormous global forces will seem fanciful, it is worth recalling the words of Primo Levi, writing about what must have seemed an equally impossible task, the struggle by groups of resistance fighters during the Second World War against the initially overwhelming successful forces of totalitarianism. The resistance fighters were motivated by a colourful range of ideologies but underlying their struggle against what must have seemed insuperable odds was the eloquent idea, so beautifully described by Levi 'If not us, who – if not now, when?' (Levi 2000).

The range of global health threats demands a similar response from health professionals, although the circumstances are more complex. Whilst Levi's guerrilla fighters could see through the supposed benefits of the totalitarian regimes against which they struggled, as we have already noted, the underlying processes which contribute to global health problems are more obscure. Take, for instance, globalization of the economy. For around 60 per cent of those living in the rich countries there have been clear financial benefits from economic globalization. But health requires societies in which all can lead lives that are emotionally, intellectually, economically, and spiritually fulfilled. Both absolute and relative poverty are closely linked to poor health. So is the lack of participatory engagement in society and the pollution which results from consumer lifestyles. Health professionals must measure the overall impact of economic globalization, including the consequences of the unregulated growth in consumption, that underpins economic globalization, which has aggravated poverty, decreased the level of participatory engagement, and provoked increasing pollution.

In their everyday work, health professionals see both the springs and neaps of these global tides. They see how greater mobility and increasing income bring many advantages to those fortunate enough to be the economic beneficiaries of the process. But they also see the impact of increasing poverty, both absolute and relative, spilling into despair, depression, and violence for the majority of the world's peoples. They are confronted by the diseases of uprooted communities, such as acquired immune deficiency syndrome (AIDS) and tuberculosis, as well as by the diseases acquired by the newly affluent tourists. They see the despoilation of the environment, and hear the anger of those suffering from atmospheric and noise pollution, as well as the joys of those newly liberated by the unparalleled ability of the affluent billion to travel as and where they please. They hear of the increasing ferocity of hurricanes, oceanic current changes, and droughts, affecting mainly the already impoverished, and wait in trepidation for the consequences of climate change to tear through the fabric of society. The rich benefit from their ability to eat any food at any time in any place, but many now worry at the as yet unquantified health implications of the persistent organic pollutants which make this possible, yet which are accumulating in food chains. Consumer societies, which make possible the food revolution, and form the basis for one of the great health advances of the century, the increasing life span of 2 billion people, are also the engines of climate change.

Health professionals are used to dealing with these types of complexity, as in their everyday work they explain complex problems to all manner of people. Individuals still trust them to a greater extent than any other social group outside of the family. Furthermore in most affluent societies, over 90 per cent of people have contact with a health professional in most years of their lives, and many health professionals are in a position to influence national and international organizations.

Health professionals thus have a unique combination of competence in communication, trust of civil society, intimate contact with most of the members thereof, and the capacity to influence individuals whatever their role in society. Like the Second World War resistance movements, they have no common ideology, but are all committed to the health of their individual patients, their communities, and their globe. However, many lack the knowledge and the inspiration through example, to live up to Primo Levi's injunction. This book seeks to offer these things.

References

Bouma, M. J., Kovats, R. S., Goubet, S. A. *et al.* (1997) Global assessment of El Niño's disaster burden. *Lancet,* **350,** 1435–8.

Davies, N. (1999) *The isles.* Macmillan, London.

Davis, M. (2001) *Late Victorian holocausts: El Niño famines and the making of the third world.* Verso, London.

Diamond, J. (1997) *Guns, germs and steel.* Jonathan Cape, London.

Fidler, D. (1999) *International law on infectious diseases.* Clarendon Press, Oxford.

Goodman, N. (1971) *International health organizations and their work.* Churchill Livingstone, Edinburgh.

Gribbin, J. and Gribbin, M. (1990) *Children of the ice.* Basil Blackwell, Oxford

Jha, P. and Chaloupka, F. J. (1999) *Curbing the epidemic: governments and the economics of tobacco control.* World Bank, Washington DC.

Keys, D. (1999) *Catastrophe. An investigation into the origins of the modern world.* Century Books, London.

Klein, N. (1999) *No logo.* Flamingo, London.

Koivusalo, M. and Ollial, E. (1997) *Making a healthy world.* STAKES/Zed Books, Helsinki.

Leigh-Fermor, P. (1984) *The travellers tree.* Penguin, Harmondsworth.

Levi, P. (2000) *If not now, when.* Penguin, Harmondsworth.

McKee, M. and Lang, T. (1996) Secret government: the Scott report. Links with industry cast doubt on the government's role in public health. *British Medical Journal*, **312**, 455–6.

McKee, M., Lang, T., and Roberts, J. (1996) Deregulating health: policy lessons of the BSE affair. *Journal of Royal Society of Medicine*, **89**, 424–6.

McLuhan, M. and Powers, B. R. (1989) *The global village: transformations in world life and media in the 21st century.* Oxford University Press, New York.

McMichael, A. J. (2001) *Human frontiers, environments and disease: past patterns, uncertain fugures.* Cambridge University Press, Cambridge.

McNeil, W. H. (1976) *Plagues and people.* Penguin, Harmondsworth.

Murray, C. and Lopez, A. (1996) *The global burden of disease.* Harvard School of Public Health/World Bank, Cambridge, MA.

Porter, R. (1997) *The greatest benefit to mankind. A medical history of humanity from antiquity to the present.* Harper Collins, London.

Rodrik, D. (1997) *Has globalization gone too far?* Institute for International Economics, Washington DC.

Shawcross, W. (2000) *Deliver us from evil: warlords and peacekeepers in a world of endless conflict.* Bloomsbury, London.

Soros, G. (1998) *The crisis of global capitalism: open society endangered.* Little Brown, London.

Stanley, D. (2000) *South Pacific handbook.* Avalon, Emeryville, CA.

World Bank (1993) *Investing in health.* Oxford University Press, New York.

Young, L. B. (1983) *The blue planet.* Little Brown, Boston.

Postman, N., Weingartner, C: *Teaching as a subversive activity.* New York: Dell, 1969.

Chapter 2

Globalization – a new agenda for health?

Kelley Lee

Introduction

The widespread recognition of the need to better understand, and respond effectively to, the challenges that a globalizing world is creating for human health is beginning to bear fruit with efforts to define a new agenda for global health. These efforts have come from far and wide. From the political right, globalization is seen as an essentially progressive force driven by high technology and economic liberalization (Ohmae 1995). Technological advances and economic growth are eventually expected to bring health benefits for all in an increasingly interdependent world. From the political left, in contrast, globalization is unfettered capitalism writ large, threatening to undermine health for all (Martin and Schumann 1996). From the developing world, where evidence of worsening health inequalities are most starkly apparent, there are concerns that globalization is a further manifestation of the dominance of wealthy countries (Chossudovsky 1997). Within the corridors of power in richer countries, however, global health is cast in terms of threats from new and re-emerging diseases; or it is played up as a golden opportunity to exploit new markets for health goods and services (Institutes of Medicine 1997).

These varied, and at times contradictory, perspectives on global health are a testament to the complex nature of globalization. There is no doubt that there are many different spins on globalization and health depending on one's political stripe, economic interest, gender, geographical location, and disciplinary background. With globalization meaning so many things to so many people, setting a new agenda for global health that will satisfy all is a daunting and perhaps futile task indeed. It is not the purpose of this chapter, therefore, to present a vision of consensus.

The starting point for this chapter, and this book, is that something broadly called globalization is happening, and that this process is raising new challenges for health. Foremost is a need to understand what is essentially 'new' about globalization and how it is creating distinct impacts. The chapter begins by describing a conceptual framework that defines globalization as a process of change affecting human societies across a range of spheres and along three dimensions – spatial, temporal, and cognitive. Each of these dimensions is briefly examined in relation to some of the potential impacts on health.

From this conceptual framework, we begin to identify an agenda that addresses four key gaps – jurisdiction, participation, incentive and knowledge. The first three are policy-oriented in their aims, processes, and outcomes, while the last concerns the strengthening of global health research. While the challenge to address these gaps will need to be taken up by a constituency of unprecedented breadth and diversity, this chapter focuses on the critical role of health professionals in moving forward this new agenda for global health.

Globalization in historical perspective: old and new?

One of the key debates surrounding globalization is whether there is anything distinctly new or whether it is in fact 'old wine in new bottles'. Sceptics doubt that there is anything qualitatively different happening or they reserve their judgement that what is happening is not historically significant (Hirst and Thompson 1996). Globalists, however, argue that there is a major transformation occurring across almost all societies, changing the way we organize ourselves and interact together. Among the most ardent globalists are those who see globalization as a recent phenomenon dating from the late twentieth century, give or take a decade or so. Technological developments in communications and transportation, in particular, are cited as hurtling the world towards unprecedented interconnectedness. Changes in production systems and corporate management are also giving rise to a global economy (Ohmae 1995). This transition to a global society is seen as leading to the end of the nation state and the beginning of new allegiances and identities.

These widely varying views seem, in large part, to be influenced by timeframe. A useful historical perspective for understanding what is both old and new about globalization is offered by Robertson (1992). He writes that the origins of globalization, as it is currently manifesting itself, lie in the fourteenth century and the age of European exploration. This dating of globalization does not ignore the widespread interaction of non-European peoples prior to this date. The Mongol Empire and trade along the silk route, for example, had clear impacts on patterns of human health. However, Robertson seeks to trace the historical origins of twentieth century globalization, a globalization dominated by western capitalist countries and large corporations.

Five stages of globalization have followed, each characterized by the development of particular technologies, spread of certain ideas and practices, and migration of peoples. Over the last five centuries there has been a gradual intensification of flows of people, accompanied by changes to the composition and organization of human societies. From the 1960s, globalization reached a period of uncertainty with *inter alia* the encompassing of the developing world, the end of the Cold War, accelerating environmental degradation and, above all, the ineffectiveness of existing institutions to achieve international cooperation. In this sense, globalization today is distinct in the intensity of human interaction taking place and the uncertain context in which it is occurring.

Whatever the nuances of dating globalization, a timeframe of centuries rather than decades fits well with historical patterns of human health. On the history of communicable disease, for example, the arrival of Christopher Columbus in the Americas in 1492 is identified by medical historians as the prelude to an unprecedented exchange of infectious agents across continents. With the flourishing of the slave trade, and later coloniz-ation of many parts of Asia, Africa, and Latin America, diseases such as measles, plague, smallpox, poliomyelitis, yaws, filariasis, and malaria were spread (Crosby 1972; McNeill 1976; Cohen 1989). Similarly, changes in human nutrition can be dated from the intro-duction of new crops (for example maize and wheat) to different parts of the world, different farming practices, and growth in intercontinental trade. Furthermore, patterns of industrialization and urbanization are closely related to the epidemiology of many human diseases such as tuberculosis and cholera. Globalization therefore, must be 'embedded in. . .social and political history', as Roemer (1994) writes, a history that scholars are only beginning to piece together.

Recognizing the historical context of globalization and health, the focus of current policy interest in global health can be located within Robertson's 'uncertainty phase'. As described above, this period is distinct in the intensity of human interaction tak-ing place and the uncertain context faced. More specifically, we can define *globaliz-ation* as a process of change affecting human interaction across a range of spheres including the economic, political, technological, socio-cultural, and environmental. The nature of this change is 'globalizing' in the sense that boundaries hitherto sepa-rating us from each other are being affected. These boundaries – spatial, temporal, and cognitive – can be described as the dimensions of globalization. Briefly, the *spatial dimension* concerns changes to how we perceive and experience physical space or geo-graphical territory. The *temporal dimension* concerns changes to how we perceive and experience time. The *cognitive dimension* concerns changes to how we think about ourselves and the world around us. What seems to be new about globalization from the late twentieth century is the scale, pace, and intensity of these changes as they are occurring across human societies – rich and poor, north and south, east and west. Furthermore, it is the simultaneous nature of these changes across all three dimen-sions that characterize current forms of globalization (Lee 2000).

Conceptualizing globalization as a health issue

Having clarified what we mean by globalization, as it is presently manifesting itself, we can begin conceptualizing how this complex and multi-faceted process may be impacting on human health. The linkages between globalization and health are, of course, highly diverse. Figure 2.1 illustrates these linkages in terms of globalizing forces, the drivers of globalization, and the determinants of health. The outcomes of these effects, in turn, have implications for various broad areas of health. To under-stand more specifically these potential impacts, each dimension of globalization is explored further below.

The spatial dimension: how to achieve health in a 'global village'

The *spatial dimension* of globalization concerns changes to how we perceive and experience physical space or territory. Scholte (1998) defines globalization as 'processes whereby social relations acquire relatively distanceless and borderless qualities, so that human lives are increasingly played out in the world as a single

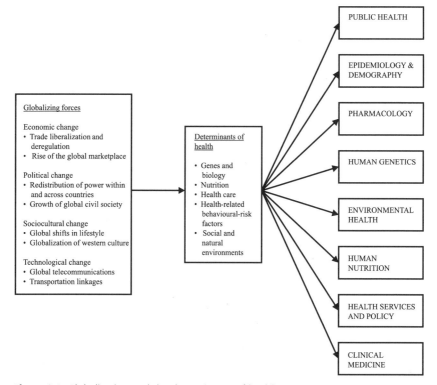

Figure 2.1 Globalization and the determinants of health

place'. This transcendence of geography lies at the heart of the concept of a global society, as distinct from an international society, defined by Fidler (1998) as 'a society made of individuals and other non-state entities all over the world that conceive of themselves as part of a single community and work nationally and transnationally to advance their common interests and values. Individuals rather than states are the key engines for global society.' Thus, the popular images of globalization as leading to the end of the nation state, and the emergence of a 'global village', stems from changes to this spatial dimension.

Importantly, the distinction between cross-border and trans-border activities is a critical one. Cross-border flows of people, goods, services, and ideas across countries have been occurring as long as sovereign states have existed (that is, since the Treaty of Westphalia of 1648). What defines globalization, however, is the intensification of trans-border activities, flows that occur with little or no regard to physical geography. Weiss (1999) refers to this as 'territorial transcendence' which does not mean, in a literal sense, that state borders are necessarily dissolving or breaking down, but that they are becoming relatively less important than other organizing principles. Thus, politically defined territories (that is, states) are being accompanied by economically (for example trans-national corporations), technologically (for example cyberspace) and environmentally (for example El Niño) defined spaces.

Global health, in this context, as opposed to *international* health, is about trans-border flows of people, goods, services, technologies, and ideas that impact upon the determinants of health. This definition of global health includes, for example, health risks arising from certain infectious diseases (Altman 1999; Porter *et al.* 1996), ozone depletion (McMichael and Haines 1997), and lifestyle changes, all of which can transcend national borders. It excludes, however, the currently limited movement of health professionals across state borders because this remains closely regulated by national authorities. The increasing cross-border transmission of food-borne diseases because of changes in patterns of food production and trade (Sanders 1999) could potentially be confined to an international health issue if the problem is effectively addressed through national regulation (for example the US Food and Drug Administration or the UK Food Standards Agency) although as Weinberg (Chapter 4) shows, this is not the case. The need to strengthen national institutions in lower-income countries in the regulation of drugs, for example, is also an international health issue (Weerasuriya 1996). However, if the skills and training of health professionals become recognized in all countries, such that there is freedom to practise unrestricted anywhere in the world, this would constitute a globalization of health professionals. Correspondingly, the public health impact of the bovine spongiform encephalopathy (BSE) crisis in the long term would become more global than international if there is an inability of national (and regional) authorities to control the infective agent through, for example, environmental contamination.

Box 2.1: **Globalization and cholera**

For centuries cholera had been confined to the riverine areas of the Indian subcontinent, with occasional outbreaks further afield as a result of trade links or religious pilgrimages. In 1826 cholera spread for the first time beyond these regions to other parts of the world. Five further pandemics followed up to the mid-1960s, with the disease spreading from country to neighbouring country in a relatively linear fashion.

The seventh cholera pandemic began in Indonesia in 1961 after a gap of 38 years. With improvements in basic sanitation, housing, and water supplies in many parts of the world, it was thought that the disease was in general decline. However, this pandemic posed new challenges. First, it was caused by a new biotype of *Vibrio cholerae* known as El Tor, less virulent but more difficult to eradicate because of a higher proportion of asymptomatic infections and greater resistance to antibiotics and chlorine. Second, El Tor cholera spread to an unprecedented number of countries, many of which had never experienced the disease before or had thought it had been long eradicated. Countries with weak public health systems, as a consequence of economic or political instability, were especially vulnerable. Third, the

Box 2.1: **Globalization and cholera** *(continued)*

disease 'hopped' continents via aeroplanes and ships, thus spreading to countries not neighbouring other affected countries. Finally, the pandemic spread at an unprecedented rate because of the above features, posing a serious and persistent challenge for public health systems.

Source: Lee and Dodgson 2000

In short, the spatial dimension of globalization represents a challenge to health professionals to shift their mental map of the world. Rather than defining health in terms of the primacy of the state and national health systems, global health requires a vision of the world as comprising individuals moving and interacting within a global society. Individuals come together collectively as states, but also demonstrate other characteristics defined by socio-economic group, ethnic origin, profession, gender, age, degree of mobility, level of technological literacy, and so on. The global health picture, in other words, offers up many images of the world and will require imaginative ways of understanding and responding to these alternative parameters.

With the rise of trans-border health risks, state-defined methods for measuring health and disease need to be reassessed. Important work has been done to improve the quality of information about patterns of disease across all countries (Murray and Lopez 1996), but much remains to be done to strengthen capacity in poorer countries. Nonetheless, a truly global picture of the burden of disease will be more than aggregates of national and regional figures. Nor is global health the same as comparative health studies (Freeman *et al.* 1995; Roemer 1994). Globalization appears to be leading to patterns of health and disease that cut across countries and regions, creating new spatial configurations that are not necessarily captured by existing data. These trans-border patterns may reveal, for example, common health needs in certain social groups within Southeast Asian, Latin American and eastern European countries as a consequence of the global economic crises of the late 1990s. Similarly, more affluent populations in many middle-income countries may have health needs that are closer in profile to wealthier populations in higher-income countries than fellow citizens in their own countries.

The temporal dimension

One of the key features of globalization has been how the process is changing the ways in which we perceive and experience time. In large part, globalization is accelerating our lives so that we are moving, doing, and experiencing life faster than we have ever done before. Technological changes have enabled us, for example, to invest our money, send e-mails, shop on-line, and be entertained twenty-four hours a day. The speed that we have come to expect from our computers, household appliances, and transport systems moves ever forward in line with the intensification of our daily lives.

This increasingly frenetic pace of life, crammed full with work and play, raises profound implications for health. On an individual level, changes to our lifestyles as a result of globalizing forces may be contributing to rising levels of coronary heart disease, high blood pressure, mental illness, and other stress-related conditions (Box 2.2). But it may also be offering us time-saving devices that lead to increasing opportunities for leisure and relaxation.

On a collective level, the acceleration of human activity poses a range of challenges for public health. The most obvious is the more rapid spread of communicable disease across national borders of which there are many examples including cholera (see Box 2.1), HIV/AIDS and tuberculosis. One example that has so far received less scholarly attention has been influenza. Detailed global analysis of influenza pandemics over many centuries is hindered by a lack of historical data on mortality and morbidity, the rapidly changing nature of the infectious agent, and seasonal differences in disease patterns. Nonetheless, it is a useful disease for analysing the extent to which globalisation may be influencing the epidemiology of communicable diseases. Historically, influenza has always moved as fast as people could, travelling across continents over a number of weeks and months. As Patterson (1986) writes,

> At no time did the rate of spread exceed the speed of human travel, which for most of the period was by food, horse, or sail. Influenza was, of course, spread much more rapidly in 1889 than ever before, through railroad and steamship travel. The pandemics of 1791 and 1830 moved at a more leisurely pace than the others.

In an age of air travel, the worldwide spread of influenza has accelerated from weeks and months, to a few days. The acceleration of this public health risk raises profound implications for health systems worldwide, especially if a more lethal strain of the virus arises in the future.

The increase in drug resistance, at a pace faster than the time needed to develop new drugs, is also widely linked to globalizing forces, notably the liberalization of trade in pharmaceuticals and accompanying poor regulation of prescribing practices. Drug-resistant forms of diseases include malaria, mycobacterium tuberculosis, neisseria gonorrhoeae, streptococcus pneumonia, and meningitis. Patterns of anti-microbial resistance also suggest close connections with globalization. From the emergence of the first forms of resistance to penicillin in the late 1940s, to the accelerating fall of the anti-microbial arsenal over the next five decades, the time available to develop new drugs has become shorter and shorter. By 1996 the appearance of the so-called 'superbug', multi-drug resistant *Staphylococcus aureus* (MRSA), signalled that bacteria were catching up and levelling the playing field once again. More important, however, has been the substantial over and misuse of drugs worldwide, and the threat of the resulting resistance spreading through greater human mobility (O'Brien 1997). As such,

> . . .antibiotic resistance is a global and social problem. Even if an individual scrupulously follows antibiotic regimens and uses them sparingly, he or she is still vulnerable to resistant strains that have emerged anywhere in the world. And with air travel and international commerce shrinking the global village, no place is safe. . .The next wave of bugs is just a few days away.

(Fred Tenover, Chief of CDC Nosocomial Pathogens
Laboratory Branch as quoted in Stolberg (1998))

Interestingly, the image of contagion has also been used to describe the rapid knock-on effects that the global economic crisis of the late 1990s has had on countries around the world. Beginning in Southeast Asia, panic among financial investors and speculators spread the crises rapidly to other parts of Asia, Latin America, and Eastern Europe. Eventually, the financial crisis reached western Europe and North America. The impact of the crisis on the social sector of affected countries illustrated the close link between the health of the global economy and the health of populations. A study by the United Nations Population Fund (1998) observed significant declines in public expenditure on health in Indonesia, Thailand, Malaysia, and the Philippines following the crisis. Empirical research of this kind remains limited, with economic policy and trade negotiations largely focusing on how liberalization of trade can be 'fast tracked' to speed the global exchange of goods and services. Public health regulations are seen largely as a hindrance to smoother trade, and concerted efforts are currently being made to find points of agreement between the trade and health agendas (Houriet 1998; World Health Organization (WHO) 1998; World Trade Organization (WTO) 1998).

As well as an acceleration of timeframes, there are concerns that some of the impacts of globalization may be longer term and even irreversible. The controversy over genetically modified (GM) foods, for example, is over the potential impact that such technologies could have in the medium and long term including across generations. If GM technology proves a danger to human health and the environment, the effects may be impossible to reverse for a very long time. The application of the so-called 'precautionary principle', whereby a more cautious approach to the use of the technology is taken despite a current lack of recognized scientific evidence because of the serious widespread and long-term impacts, is based on this weighing up of potential risks and benefits.

As well as affecting the speed with which certain health risks are arising, globalizing forces can also offer opportunities for speeding our responses to them. Most prominent are the capabilities of modern technologies for information collection and dissemination, which offer a multitude of applications that are only beginning to be explored. For example, efforts are underway to improve the surveillance, monitoring, and reporting systems of infectious diseases (Chapter 4), the health effects of global climate change (Chapter 5) and anti-microbial resistance (for example WHONET database software for the management of microbiology laboratory data and the analysis of antimicrobiol susceptibility test results). The latter requires improved data on anti-bacterial susceptibility patterns which, if regularly disseminated to prescribers, would improve the empirical selection of anti-microbial agents, help to develop treatment guidelines, and provide prompt treatment with newer agents to combat resistance (Fasehun 1999). The speed and reach of new technologies could also be used to extend health education and training (for example distance-based learning) to build the global capacity of public health professionals notably in lower-income countries.

Thus, global health concerns changes to the timeframe that health risks and opportunities manifest themselves. The key challenge for health professionals will be to recognize how their work must be adopted accordingly, what institutional changes may be necessary, and whether effective responses can be achieved by taking advantage of available technologies.

Box 2.2: **The health effects of life as Type A**

The term 'Type A personality' was coined by cardiologists Meyer Friedman and Ray Rosenman in the late 1950s to describe individuals who have a tendency to be excessively impatient, competitive, aggressive, and high-achieving. They believed that living life as a race against the clock has adverse effects on health in the form of raised blood pressure, coronary heart disease, and mental stress. An entire industry subsequently has evolved to treat 'hurry sickness' through yoga, meditation, counselling, and relaxation tapes.

Three decades of research on the Type A personality, however, has failed to produce any carefully specified and measurable set of character traits that predict heart disease, or to demonstrate that people who change their behaviour will lower their health risks. The reason is not that these traits do not exist but that they are increasingly apparent in the behaviour of so many people because of changes in lifestyle. In other words, it is not a particular character trait but a particular lifestyle trait that we are all increasingly sharing. In a world of fast-food drive-throughs, instant credit, multi-tasking, power walking, hypermarkets, and speed dialling, we are moving at an ever-increasing pace through our lives because we can and therefore we do.

Source: Gleick 1999

The cognitive dimension

The cognitive dimension of globalization concerns changes to how we see ourselves and the world around us. It encompasses a broad range of thought processes, from the creation of knowledge and experiences, to their dissemination and application for practical purposes. The cognitive dimension is especially central to health. In so many ways, health is influenced, pursued, and promoted by the way we think; for example, as a precursor to health-seeking behaviour, as a basis for health interventions and clinical treatment, and as the primary product of health research. Hence, any health system is built on a variety of cognitive processes – health education and information, training of health professionals, clinical guidelines and nomenclature, international laws and regulations, health research, and policies.

The implications of globalization for the cognitive dimension lie in the ways in which globaliszing forces are changing the way we think. Foremost is the impact of information and communication technologies that have created, at least in principle, a global network that enables us to generate ideas and share them with the world for good and bad. The potentially positive benefits stem from new avenues for the exchange of knowledge (for example adverse reactions to drugs, health information, and education), training of health professionals (for example distance-based learning), creation of global data sets, surveillance, and monitoring systems, clinical practice (for example telemedicine) and trans-border health activism (for example campaigning). Innovative use of such technologies has also led, for example, to 'virtual conferencing' that enables widely dispersed delegates to participate in a conference in real time. Many of these applications are especially promising for health systems with serious resource constraints (Robert 1999).

However, there are also profound concerns that the cognitive dimension of global health may mean an extension of ideas originating from a dominant policy elite to health systems worldwide (Box 2.3). While globalization has the potential to pluralize the health policy environment, the strongest critics see globalization as a 'closed shop' of core international organizations (for example the World Bank, the International Monetary Fund (IMF), bilateral aid agencies, management consultancy firms, leading academic institutions, and increasingly, trans-national corporations and wealthy individuals. There have been concerns, in particular, regarding the growing role of the World Bank in the health sector since the 1980s (Buse and Walt 1998). Suspicions of the cognitive influence of this new policy elite are based on recent experience of the impact that policies such as structural adjustment have had

Box 2.3: **The globalization of health care financing reform**

Health care financing is a broad term that refers to the mobilization and use of financial resources in the health sector. It encompasses both resource generation (that is, the source and mechanisms employed to raise finance), as well as the means of resource allocation and financial flows. Policy reforms to health care financing began to be introduced in higher-income countries, notably in the USA in the late 1970s as part of broader trends towards reducing public expenditure. By the early 1990s, health care financing reform had spread to much of the world with the introduction of alternative or complementary means to generate resources for health. The leading policies to achieve this were user fees and health insurance schemes.

The conduit for the globalization of health care financing reform has been a policy network of key international organizations, bilateral aid agencies, consultancy firms, and academic institutions. The global influence of this network, over both the underlying principals that should guide health care finance and the mechanisms for pursuing them, can be traced to key policy documents, meetings, and initiatives. Among these are three concurrent projects funded by the United States Agency for International Development (USAID) USAID and carried out by consultancy firms: two key World Bank publications, *Financing health services in developing countries: an agenda for reform* (1987) and *World development report, investing in health* (1993); and individual and institutional linkages between academic institutions in the USA and the UK and the developing world. This network has been reinforced through a range of formal and informal linkages. The result has been a trans-border flow of policy reforms, originating within a relatively small but highly influential policy elite, and extending outwards to strongly influence policy thinking worldwide.

Source: Lee and Goodman forthcoming

on the poor within societies. Of equal concern is the 10/90 gap, in which 90 per cent of research funds address the health needs of 10 per cent of the world's population. This reflects a failure of health research to address the needs of the majority of the world's population (Global Forum for Health Research 1999), the lack of invest-ment by private pharmaceutical companies in tropical diseases, and the priority funding by donor agencies to family planning and selected communicable diseases. Thus, among the 1223 new chemical entities commercialized from 1975–97, only 13 (one per cent) were for tropical diseases (Pecoul *et al.* 1999).

Thus, global health concerns the trans-border flow of ideas, values, policies, guidelines, nomenclature, research, and other thought processes concerned with health. The challenge for health professionals lies in balancing the capacity for global knowledge, strategies, and leadership to tackle the most pressing health issues with the equally important and particular needs of individuals and local communities.

A new global health agenda

The purpose of this chapter has been to establish what we mean by globalization and, in turn, what is new about a global health agenda. This chapter argues that there is indeed a profound shift underway from *international* to *global* health, and that understanding and responding effectively to these processes of change is unlike-ly to be achieved by 'business as usual'. The three dimensions of global health change are:

+ an increase in trans-border health risks and opportunities
+ an acceleration of the timeframe in which health risks and opportunities arise and must be addressed
+ an intensification of trans-border flows of thought processes that affect health involving a different range of actors.

While recognizing that there are opportunities from the above changes for protecting and promoting health that are only beginning to be explored, the search to define a global health agenda has so far focused on health risks. Aside from rather alarmist literature, there is a broad base of serious concern that current forms of globalization are adversely impacting on population health. Indeed, critics from different ends of the political spectrum argue that there is a distinctly unhealthy quality to contemporary globalization. They are united in their fears that a globalizing world is creating conditions for major public health risks including deteriorating health systems, increasing inequality within and across countries, growing levels of absolute poverty, weak or unregulated pollution of the natural environment, irresponsible use of antibiotics, proliferation of the illicit drug trade, threats from biological and chemical warfare, and prolonged conflict in many parts of the world fuelled by a legal and illegal arms trade. Consequently, there is already strong consensus that a global health agenda must address these concerns.

How to articulate and prioritize this complex and crowded policy agenda is the foremost task. To begin, we can draw on broader scholarly and policy debates that are rethinking many of the fundamental premises underlying international relations. Foremost has been a re-evaluation of the concept of security, beyond the traditional focus on military threats, following the end of the Cold War. Despite hopes of a 'new world order' of greater peace and security, the superpower rivalry has been replaced in the minds of high-level policy makers by non-military threats, many of which are trans-border in nature and impact. Ullman (1995) suggests an expanded definition of national security as

> ... an action or sequence of events that (1) threatens drastically and over a relatively brief span of time to degrade the quality of life for the inhabitants of a state, or (2) threatens significantly to narrow the range of policy choices available to the government of a state or to private, non-governmental entities (persons, groups, corporations) within the state.

This blurring of individual, national, and global security has led to a reassessment of policies since the 1980s that have reduced the role of the state. While debate has continued as to the appropriate size and specific roles that the state should play, the necessity for the state to provide certain 'public goods' is now an accepted one (World Bank 1997).

This search for a 'more effective state' at the national level is mirrored at the global level by discussions of the need for improved governance. Governance can be defined as the 'ability to promote collective action and deliver collective solutions' (Dodgson *et al.* 2001). As distinct from government, governance can be fulfilled by a varied range of individuals and institutions including the public sector, private companies, non-governmental organizations, professional bodies, and labour unions. This is particularly apt at the global level where sovereign states remain the dominant, but by no means the only important, actor. As Reinicke (1998) argues, the challenge lies in 'governing without government':

> Without a greater effort to understand the origin and nature of the current global transformation and its implications for public policy, we will continue to react to events rather than act to shape the future course of world politics. Such passivity will leave our societies vulnerable to the gains that a more active policymaking could realise.

Similarly, Kaul *et al.* (1999) point to the central importance of global governance for managing the externalities being created by a globalizing world. The costs and benefits of globalization are trans-border and, as such, require effective policy mechanisms to address them. Global public goods are 'goods whose benefits reach across borders, generations, and population groups'. Conversely, global 'bads' are costs that are borne collectively.

Health has been at the intersection of many of these conceptual discussions. For instance, emerging and re-emerging diseases are often cast as a potential threat to national security that requires investments in national and global health development (Institutes of Medicine 1997; Nakajima 1997). Debates about the role of the state have been central to health sector reform since the 1980s. The increased influence of the World Bank in health policy has given rise to discussion of the need for a new institutional architecture for global health – global health governance – to manage the risks and opportunities being created by globalization.

All of this suggests that the emerging global health agenda requires a strategy that brings together these emerging debates to address the distinct nature of globalization. It requires a clear research and policy agenda directed at gaps in what we know and how to put this knowledge into practice.

Kaul *et al.* (1999) identify three gaps in the current arrangements for providing global public goods that can be usefully used to help define such an agenda. The first, the **jurisdictional gap** is the discrepancy between a globalized world and national, separate units of policy making. What makes *global* health different from *international* health? For global health, this requires a mental leap in thinking about the determinants of health on many levels – local, national, regional, international, and global. Health has traditionally been understood in terms of individuals, and health systems in terms of nation states. Research and policy is largely geared to these units of analysis. Health statistics, for example, where available are primarily collected and aggregated by country but not across countries. Global health calls for an enhancement, rather than replacement, of these perspectives to incorporate trans-border impacts on health. A safe and healthy diet, for example, is about what an individual eats from day to day, but it is also about how that food is produced within a globalizing food industry. Stronger national or regional regulation of food safety and standards may effectively address current fears over food safety, but inadequately address environmental effects of GM foods or the impoverishment of small farmers by a global agribusiness.

The jurisdictional gap is also manifested in the entrenched nature of many traditional cognitive boundaries within the health field, as well as between health and other fields. The fragmentation of health professions into many specialties, such that a single individual focuses narrowly on their local patch or sub-field, does not encourage a global perspective. Furthermore, global health requires a widening of what might be shaping the determinants of health – biological and chemical weapons, terrorism, illicit drug trade, and environmental degradation. How does one incorporate these unconventional subjects? Thus, this gap requires a reflexive approach that questions how we define, measure, and promote health. What new patterns of health can we observe? How is globalization affecting the determinants of health? What intellectual and institutional boundaries need to be crossed to address global health issues?

Second, there is a *participation gap* in that health co-operation is still primarily an intergovernmental process with other actors participating on the fringes. The trans-border nature of the issues raised, however, strongly suggests that governments alone cannot address them effectively. A key challenge for the global health agenda will be to explore new forms of governance that enable a broader constituency of individuals, including health professionals, and institutions to meaningfully contribute. This may be achieved by building alliances to other sectors (for example environment) from which lessons could be learned (Fidler 2001). The building of new alliances across traditional boundaries (for example public–private partnerships) also needs to be pursued and critically assessed. Thus, the participation gap is essentially concerned with strengthening health governance at many levels. Who should be part of a system of global health governance? How would they meaningfully participate in this system? What would such a system look like and how could it created?

Third, there is an *incentive gap* in the form of an over-reliance on aid and voluntary action to achieve global public goods. The global health agenda will need to demonstrate that co-operation is the preferred option, and to identify shared interests that will motivate diverse stakeholders. This means putting global health onto the table of 'high politics' as well as the mainstream consciousness of the general public. In the USA global health has been framed as a threat to the vital interests of the USA in order to secure political leverage (Institutes of Medicine 1997). The subsequent chapters of this book could be used to make a convincing case elsewhere. There is the challenge, therefore, of framing the global health challenge appropriately and effectively to secure the political and economic resources needed to address this new agenda.

Conclusion

We are increasingly recognizing that globalization is a complex process that is having varied impacts on individuals, communities, countries, regions, and the world as a whole. In some ways, the process is putting a global 'spin' on already familiar health challenges – infectious diseases, socio-economic inequalities, and resource constraints on health financing and service provision. Where globalization is worsening existing health risks, there is already substantial evidence that should be brought together with non-health analyses of globalization. Research on the impacts of structural adjustment programmes, the pros and cons of health sector aid, and activities of pharmaceutical and tobacco companies, for example, offers crucial pieces to the puzzle of understanding globalization. At the same time, globalization is creating new challenges that spill over national borders – antibiotic resistance, environmental degradation, the illicit drug trade, and the proliferation of information technologies. Where globalization is having distinct effects, because of the trans-border nature of its impacts, there is need for new research methods and analysis, to which health professionals have much to contribute. The specifics of such research could, for instance, use Fig. 2.1 as a starting point for understanding specific linkages between globalizing forces and the determinants of health.

Acknowledgements

The author would like to thank Richard Dodgson, David Fidler, and David Sanders for providing important insights into the development of the ideas behind this paper.

References

Altman, D. (1999) Globalisation political economy, and HIV/AIDS. *Theory and Society*, **28**, 559–84.

Buse, K. and Walt, G. (2000) Role conflict? The World Bank and the world's health. *Social Science and Medicine*, **50**(2), 177–79.

Chossudovsky, M. (1997) *The globalisation of poverty, impacts of IMF and World Bank reforms.* Zed Books, London.

Cohen, M. N. (1989) *Health and the rise of civilization.* Yale University Press, New Haven.

Crosby, A. (1972) *The Columbian exchange: biological and cultural consequences of 1492.* Westport.

Dodgson, R. Conn. Lee K. and Drager N. (2000) Global health governance: a conceptual review. Greenwood Press, In *Global Health Governance: Key Issues*, ed. K. Lee. WHO Department of Health in Sustainable Development, Geneva.

Fasehun, F. (1999) The antibacterial paradox: essential drugs, effectiveness, and cost. *Bulletin of the World Health Organization*, **77**(3), 211–6.

Fidler, D. (1998) Microbialpolitick infectious diseases and international relations. *American University International Law Review*, **14**(1), 1–53.

Freeman, P., Gomez-Dantes, O., and Frenk, J. (ed.) (1995) *Health systems in an era of globalization challenges, opportunities for North America.* Institute of Medicine/Mexican National Academy of Medicine, Washington DC.

Goodman, H. and Lee, K. (2001) Global health governance: mechanisms and lessons for health. Global Health Governance Series, Discussion Paper No. 2. WHO Department of Health in Sustainable Development, Geneva.

Gleick, J. (1999). *Faster, the acceleration of just about everything.* Little Brown, New York.

Global Forum for Health Research (1999) The 10/90 report on health research. WHO, Geneva.

Hirst, P. and Thompson, G. (1996) *Globalization in question: the international economy and the possibilities of governance.* Polity Press, Cambridge.

Houriet, S. (1998) The effects of international trade liberalization on the health of poorest population groups: annotated bibliography. WHO Task Force on Health Economics, Geneva.

Institutes of Medicine (1997) *America's vital interest in global health.* National Academy Press, Washington DC.

Kaul, I., Grunberg, I., and Stern, M. (1999) *Global public goods, international cooperation in the 21st century.* Oxford University Press, Oxford.

Lee, K. (2000) Globalization and health policy: a review of the literature and proposed research and policy agenda. In *Health development in the new global economy.* Pan American Health Organization, Washington DC.

Lee, K. and Dodgson, R. (2000) Globalization and cholera: implications for global governance. *Global governance.* Overview of the role of international law in protecting and promoting global public health, ed. K. Lee, WHO Department of Health in Sustainable Development, Geneva. **6**(2) 227–8.

Lee, K. and Goodman, H. (forthcoming) Global policy networks: the propagation of health care financing reforms since the 1980s. In *Health policy in a globalising world*, ed. K. Lee, (S. Fustukian) Buse, K. Cambridge University Press, Cambridge.

Martin, H. P. and Schumann, H. (1996) *The global trap, globalization and the assault on democracy and prosperity.* Zed Books, London.

McMichael, A. J. and Haines, A. (1997) Global climate change: the potential effects on health. *British Medical Journal,* **315,** 805–9.

McNeill, W. H. (1976) *Plagues and peoples.* Basil Blackwell, Oxford.

Murray, C. and Lopez, A. (1996) *The global burden of disease.* Harvard School of Public Health/World Bank, Cambridge, MA.

Nakajima, H. (1997) Global disease threats and foreign policy. *Brown Journal of World Affairs,* **4,** 319–27.

O'Brien, T. (1997) The global epidemic nature of antimicrobial resistance and the need to manage it locally. *Clinical Infectious Disease,* **24,** S2–8.

Ohmae, K. (1995) *The end of the nation state.* Free Press, New York.

Patterson, K. D. (1986) *Pandemic influenza 1700–1900, a study in historical epidemiology.* Rowman & Littlefield, New Jersey.

Pecoul, B., Chirac, P., Trouiller, P. *et al.* (1999) Access to essential drugs in poor countries, a lost battle? *Journal of the American Medical Association,* **281**(4), 361–7.

Porter, J., Lea, G., and Caroll, B. (1996) HIV/AIDS and international travel: a global perspective? In *Health and the international tourist,* ed. S. Clift and S. Page, pp. 68–86. Routledge, London.

Reinicke, W. H. (1998) *Global public policy, governing without government?* Brookings Institution, Washington DC.

Robert, G. (1999) Science and technology, trends and issues forward to 2015: implications for health care. In *Policy futures for UK health 1999,* Technical Series. The Nuffield Trust, London/Judge Institute of Management Studies, University of Cambridge, Cambridge.

Robertson, R. (1992) *Globalization: social theory and global culture.* Sage, London.

Roemer, M. (1994) Internationalism in medicine and public health. In *The history of public health and the modern state,* ed. D. Porter, pp. 403–23. Editions Rodopi, Amsterdam.

Sanders, T. (1999) Food production and food safety. *British Medical Journal,* **318,** 1689–93.

Scholte, J. A. (1998) Food production and food safety. In *The globalization of world politics, an introduction to international relations,* ed. J. Baylis and S. Smith, pp. 13–30. Oxford University Press, Oxford.

Stolberg, S. G. (1998) Superbugs, the bacteria antibiotics can't kill. *The New York Times Magazine,* 2 August, 42–7.

Ullman, R. H. (1995) Redefining security. In *Global dangers, changing dimensions of international security,* ed. S. M. Lynn-Jones and S. E. Miller, pp. 15–39. MIT Press, Cambridge.

United Nations Population Fund (1998) Southeast asian populations in crisis, challenges to the implementation of the ICPD programme of action. UNFPA, New York/Australian National University, Canberra.

Weerasuriya, K. (1996) Globalisation of drug regulation and drug regulators in developing countries. *International Journal of Risk and Safety in Medicine,* **9**(3), 187–94.

Weiss, L. (1999) Globalization and national governance: antimonies or interdependence? *Review of International Studies,* **25,** 59–88.

WHO (1998) Food safety and the globalization of trade in food, a challenge to the public health sector. Food Safety Unit, Geneva.

World Bank (1997) World development report, the state in a changing world. IBRD, Washington DC.

WTO (1998) Health and Social Services, background note by the Secretariat. Council for Trade in Services, Doc. S/C/W/50, Geneva 18 September.

Chapter 3

The globalization of health care

Julio Frenk, Octavio Gómez-Dantés, Orvill
Adams, and Emmanuela E. Gakidou

Introduction

Change and complexity are the signs of our time. Rapid growth in international trade
and the communications revolution have eroded national borders, facilitating the
transfer of goods, services, people, ideas, values, and lifestyles from one country to
another.

The new shape of the world is reflected in the health field. Countries must confront
a vast array of challenges in order to make their health systems meet population needs.
To the internal forces that determine those challenges, national societies must now
add a series of phenomena at the global level. Chen and colleagues point to 'an era of
global "health interdependence", the health parallel to economic interdependence'
(Chen *et al.* 1996).

This complex health scenario threatens to exceed the control of national health
systems and has created an emerging demand for new forms of international co-operation. National governments still retain responsibility for the health of their populations, but they have limited control over many of the determinants of health conditions that arise from interactions at the global level.

The resources and services used to respond to health needs are also being produced
and traded through global processes that frequently transcend the regulatory capacity of individual governments. In addition, the global medical industry confronts a
bewildering array of regulatory practices in different countries, which often produces
a wasteful multiplication of compliance efforts on the part of these corporations.

It is in this context that we will discuss the globalization of health care. The first part
of the chapter will address the present situation of the global health order, with
emphasis on those changes that have taken place in the last half of the twentieth century and that now demand regional or global responses. On the side of health needs,
the international transfer of risks will be discussed in some detail. On the side of
health care, particular attention will be paid to the globalization of the medical industry and to the health system reform movement, which has generated opportunities for
shared learning and has created a new arena for negotiation. The second part (the core
of the chapter), will be devoted to a review of the globalization of health care. It will
not refer to international trade in pharmaceuticals and medical equipment or to
export of financial services related to health. Trade in health services will be addressed

in its four basic forms: (1) the export of services, (2) the international movement of health care consumers, (3) the international movement of health care providers, and (4) the establishment of facilities in other countries (Frenk and Gomez-Dantes 1995). This part will end with a discussion of the role of the World Trade Organization (WTO) in the field of health care.

The global health order

The profound change in disease patterns during the twentieth century has been called a 'health revolution' (World Health Organization (WHO) 1999*b*). In all countries of the world disease patterns have changed profoundly during the twentieth century. Despite significant progress in the health of people in all regions, nations are facing unprecedented challenges. Most developing countries are still struggling with the rapid pace of social, demographic, and epidemiological transformations, which have led them to experience a double burden of ill health.

These countries continue to suffer from common infections, reproductive health problems, and malnutrition, which keep infant and maternal mortality at unacceptably high levels. In addition to these problems, they also face the emerging challenges of non-communicable diseases and injuries, which already represent the main causes of death and disability in middle-income countries. To further complicate the picture, in the past three decades new diseases and variants of old diseases have been identified, and are having a major impact on epidemiological patterns in both developed and developing countries. The human immuno-deficiency virus (HIV)/acquired immune deficiency syndrome (AIDS) pandemic is the most dramatic example. The emergence of these threats, coupled with the rising resistance to drugs of major pathogens and the declining investment in research for new anti-microbials (Amyes 2000) could reverse the recent declines in mortality rates due to communicable diseases.

These transitions are being influenced by increasing trade and related phenomena. There has been a growth in international trade blocs such as the North American Free Trade Agreement (NAFTA), Mercosur (Argentina, Brazil, Paraguay, and Uruguay, with Bolivia and Chile as associates), the European Union (EU), the Association of South-East Asian Nations (ASEAN), the Southern African Development Community (SADEC) and other regional trade agreements. Together with the establishment of the WTO in 1995, this process has fuelled the debate about the benefits of more open trade and its impact on health.

The international transfer of health risks occurs as a result of six basic processes (Frenk *et al.* 1997).

(1) *The rise of global environmental threats* (Chapter 5). Due to their ability to move across borders, many environmental threats with health implications (ozone depletion, greenhouse effect) have become the common problem of rich and poor nations.

(2) *The movement of people* (Chapter 9). The growth in international trade, tourism, military conflict, and migration has intensified cross-border movement of people in recent decades, contributing to the spread of health problems.

(3) *The adoption of risky lifestyles.* The international spread of unhealthy lifestyles and diets creates further health risks, including cardiovascular diseases, obesity, and certain forms of cancer.

(4) *The variance in environmental and occupational health and safety standards.* This variance in standards between the developed and developing world also leads to serious health risks, and encourages some multi-national corporations to avoid stringent regulations in the developed world by transferring their operations to developing nations.

(5) *The trade in harmful legal and illegal products.* Tobacco produces four million deaths a year nowadays and this figure may reach 10 million by the year 2030 (see Chapter 8). Yet exports of this product in 1997 exceeded US$5 billion (Townsend 1999). Meanwhile, worldwide consumption of heroine and cocaine, also controlled through international networks, has grown 10 times in the last 20 years.

(6) *The spread of medical technologies.* Even medical technology can prove to be a health and financial risk. The best example is the spread of drug resistance as a result of inadequate antibiotic prescription. This phenomenon is creating annual costs in excess of US$4 billion in direct treatment just in the USA (Chen *et al.* 1999).

Against the backdrop of these changes, there has been a parallel growth in the complexity of the social arrangements to respond to health needs. Health care systems have expanded into a network of agencies and institutions that consume an increasingly large share of resources. In 1994, public and private expenditure on formal health services worldwide reached nine per cent of the total world product. Industrialized countries spent almost 90 per cent of this amount (Schieber and Maeda 1999). In contrast, developing countries, with 84 per cent of the world population and 92 per cent of the worldwide burden of disease, spent the remaining 10 per cent.

In developed nations, health care systems face the challenge of increasing demand associated with ageing populations and rising physician dependence on medical technology, with a resulting explosion in costs.

In developing countries, health systems are experiencing major pressures as a result of the double burden mentioned earlier. Hence, these systems must design and implement more efficient ways of delivering the cost-effective interventions that are already available to deal with the backlog of common infections, reproductive health problems, and malnutrition. At the same time, they face the additional challenge of developing or adapting affordable and effective interventions for non-communicable problems.

Recent changes in health care have been associated with an increasing globalization of the health care industry. The liberalization of global trade has expanded the international market for health products and services. Medicinal and pharmaceutical exports from the Organization for Economic Co-operation and Development (OECD) countries increased from US$6 billion in 1975 to US$52.8 billion in 1994 (OECD 1994). The export of professional and scientific instruments, an important proportion of which are medical instruments, has also increased, from US$7.8 billion in 1975 to US$59.7 billion in 1994 in this same group of countries. Medical services are also being increasingly traded through international markets as we discuss next.

The globalization of health care services

This section focuses on the globalization of health care services, without addressing alternative therapies, an emerging phenomenon, which deserves a separate discussion. Other aspects of the globalization of the health care market, such as the exportation of drugs, medical devices, and financial services (indemnity insurance) are crucial to the global health care market, but are beyond the scope of the present discussion.

International trade in health services

Health services do not escape the general process of economic globalization. As the great historian of the twentieth century, Eric Hobsbawm has written, '. . . for many purposes, notably in economic affairs, the globe is now the primary operational unit. . .' (Hobsbawm 1994).

The traditional classification of international trade in services, includes four basic forms: (1) the export of services, (2) the movement of consumers, (3) the movement of providers, and (4) the establishment of facilities in other countries (commercial presence).

Export of services

In the health field, export of services involves the movement of diagnostic methods or therapeutic procedures between health institutions or professionals in different countries. As a result of recent technological innovations in transportation and communication, export of services has increased in the last decades. The regular cross-border use of laboratory and diagnostic facilities and the development of international 'telemedicine' (teleradiology, teleconferencing, teleconsulting, mobile telemedicine testbeds, 'electronic housecalls') serve as expressions of this increase in the export of health services. WorldCare Limited, for example, with headquarters in Bermuda and access to physicians at the Massachusetts General Hospital, the Cleveland Clinic, and Johns Hopkins University, among others, has telemedicine projects in the UK, the USA, and several countries in Latin America, the Middle East, and Asia. Among the telemedicine services it provides, patient management consultation attracts the largest demand (Larkin 1997).

Movement of consumers

The movement of consumers across political boundaries in order to obtain health care services is also becoming a frequent occurrence, particularly between bordering countries. This phenomenon has often been attributed to differences in cost and quality of care, but lately, new motives have been proposed for why consumers cross political boundaries while seeking health care.

For cultural and legal reasons, organ transplants in Japan are scarce, and for regulatory reasons certain treatments are not available in Europe or North America. To this we

Table 3.1 Main opportunities and challenges arising from international trade of health services

	Equity		Efficiency		Quality	
	Opportunities	Challenges	Opportunities	Challenges	Opportunities	Challenges
Trade mechanisms export of services	• Improve access in remote areas • Ease access to locally unavailable services	• Avoid concentration of human and financial resources in high-tech activities	• Increase efficiency in the delivery of specialized services	• Discourage use of non-cost-effective interventions • Mobilize the required investment	• Enhance timeliness and quality of services	• Establish quality comparisons and regulatory mechanisms
Movement of consumers	• Improve access to an increased variety of health services	• Avoid resources skewed to care for foreigners	• Target cost-effective services and training	• Avoid resources spent on non-cost-effective services for foreign patients	• Improve quality locally to attract foreign patients	• Assure same quality to local and foreign patients

should add the existence of an emerging consumer class in developing countries. For example in the European market, European Community (EC) regulations (Leidel 1993) have stimulated the use of French health services by Northern Italians due to differences in the perceived quality of the services in these two countries.

American residents regularly use dental and ophthalmological services of Mexican border cities, which are cheaper than in the USA and are usually not covered by American insurance schemes. Australia recently introduced a 'medical visa' for people seeking health care and established specialized international departments in some of its teaching hospitals (Walt 1998). Cuba is increasingly marketing its health services to foreign visitors, generating over US$25 million in 1995 (United Nations Commission on Trade and Development (UNCTAD) 1998). Costa Rica is offering essential and elective health services through its Health Tourism Corporation. American hospitals, confronted with an oversupply of beds due to the high managed-care penetration, are prompting marketing campaigns to attract foreign patients searching for high-quality care or in need of specialized services. Johns Hopkins Medical Center, for example, recently signed contracts with Peru and Ecuador to treat soldiers wounded in local conflicts (Lagnado 1996).

The USA national accounts include the 'exportation of health services', defined as the 'hospital income generated by foreign patients travelling to the USA to get any sort of medical treatment' (OECD 1992). In 1994, income in this category totalled $US794 million – very probably an underestimation – which represents an increase of more than 100 per cent in relation to 1981 (US$352 million).

The supply of these health tourism services through the Internet – 'a major, perhaps eventually *the* major, worldwide distribution channel for goods, for services and, surprisingly, for managerial and professional jobs' (Drucker 1999) – is ubiquitous, from treatment for chronic back pain in Crimea, to traditional massage for rheumatism in Kerala, and cardiac surgery in the Swiss Alps. Global Health Systems, in fact, is already building a worldwide electronic database of health tourism providers.

Trade liberalization may favour the international mobility of health care consumers. In a recent ruling of the European Court of Justice, it was concluded that national regulations which make the reimbursement of the costs of medical treatment or medical products obtained in other member states subject to the prior authorization of sickness funds are in principle incompatible with the free movement of medical goods and services in the region and should be reviewed (Van der Mei 1999).

Movement of providers

The movement of providers across international borders has been a common phenomenon. The main exporting countries have been India and the Philippines (World Bank 1993). The Philippines alone had lost 14,000 doctors and 89,000 nurses by 1982 (Abel-Smith 1986). This 'health manpower drain' usually follows roads leading to North America and Europe – imports worth billions of dollars to the recipient nations – but recently physicians have also been hired by Gulf states and other middle eastern nations. Countries exporting nurses include Australia, Canada, the UK, Jamaica, and the Philippines. Jamaica and the UK, for example, export nurses to the USA and import them to meet local shortages from Myanmar and Nigeria, and from Ireland, the West Indies and Mauritius, respectively.

This phenomenon will probably increase, as nations from different trading blocs are harmonizing their licensing and certification criteria. Directives for harmonization between EC member states were adopted for physicians in 1975 and for nurses in 1977 (McKee *et al.* 1996). The member states of this bloc recently agreed on the recognition of a professional regional credential for physicians and are moving towards a 'European' model for graduate medical education and towards a baccalaureate prepared nurse (Boufford 1995). The North American Free Trade Agreement also contains provisions that allow the governments involved in this agreement to encourage professional groups to discuss the criteria that might eventually be applied in the region with regard to the licensing and certification of professional health service providers (Gomez-Dantes *et al.* 1997).

Most of the foreign physicians entered the US health care system through their enrolment in graduate medical education programmes. The total number of foreign physicians in training continues to increase (Forum on the Future of Academic Medicine, website).

More than 21 000 Nigerian doctors are practising in the USA (United Nations Development Programme (UNDP) 1999). The WHO health statistics (WHO 1998) showed over 250 citizens from India received fellowships for medical training in the UK and the USA in 1996–7. Between 1961 and 1983, at least 70 000 scientists, engineers, doctors, and other highly skilled people emigrated from developing countries to the USA, Canada, and the UK (International Labour Office 1994). Data on the performance of medical residents training in internal medicine in the USA showed a total number of 2903 international medical students registered to take the in-training exam in the first year of medical school (Waxman 1997).

Cross-border establishment of facilities

The cross-border establishment of health care facilities is growing at a faster pace than any other form of international exchange of personal health services. In addition to the general move of corporations towards the service sector as profitability in manufacturing declines, three current trends explain this process: (1) trade liberalization through the creation of regional trading blocs, (2) the expansion of US health care services in the international market, and (3) the nature of the health care reforms that are being implemented in many developed and developing nations.

Trade liberalization through NAFTA, for example, significantly increased US firms' interest in the Mexican health care sector. Eighty per cent of the respondents to a survey distributed to the participants in the 1994 Health Care in Mexico Conference agreed that NAFTA had favourably changed the investment horizon for conducting business in the Mexican health care sector (Gomez-Dantes and Frenk 1995). Survey respondents identified hospitals, clinics, and Health Maintenance Organisations (HMOs) as the most profitable sectors of the Mexican health care market. Not surprisingly, health care facilities financed partly or wholly by American firms were established in the Mexican cities of Aguascalientes, Mazatlán, and Tijuana in the mid–1990s (Carlino 1994).

Other countries are witnessing similar trends. Stanford University Medical Center and the Cleveland Clinic, for example, are building in-patient care sites in Singapore and Cairo, and middle eastern countries are trying to attract foreign investments to upgrade their health care infrastructure (Berlow and Trig 1997).

Private hospitals and specialty clinics, especially cardiac and cancer centres, are being built in Malaysia, Thailand, and Indonesia to prevent their patients from seeking health care in neighbouring countries. During the past five years, public and private hospitals in Kuala Lumpur have increased the number of hospital beds. Jakarta has faced a growth of 24-hour-seven-days-a-week clinics for local and foreign nationals who seek routine medical treatment. Patients are referred to Singapore when there is a need for technologically advanced equipment (Desker 1991).

Foreign companies from Australia, Malaysia, Japan, and Singapore have shown an interest in managing Indonesian hospitals. Parkway Group Healthcare, a Singaporean firm has hospitals in Jakarta, Surabaya, and Medan (Widiatmoke and Gani 1999).

In Thailand the number of private hospitals and clinics has increased from 11 495 in 1989 to 11 988 in 1994. Foreign-owned private hospitals form joint ventures (with 49 per cent of total investment) with local firms in order to operate facilities in Thailand (Widiatmoke and Gani 1999).

Additional US market forces should accelerate the trend towards increased direct foreign investment in health care. The international expansion of those US managed-care corporations who are in a position to take advantage of the opportunities offered by globalization will also be a result of saturation in the US health care market. By the year 2000, market researchers estimated that 80 per cent of the total US population would be insured by some sort of managed-care organization (Smith 1996). Given that the majority of these managed-care organizations are for-profit enterprises, they will seek out new growth markets to guarantee a 'reasonable' return for their investments when local demand stabilizes.

Due to its geographical proximity and the expectations generated by the emergence of several free trade pacts, Latin America has captured the attention of US managed-care organizations. As a continent, Latin America represents an enormous market where pre-paid, non-governmental, integrated delivery organizations already care for more than 60 million people (Medici *et al.* 1997). In Argentina, 3 million people are covered by pre-paid schemes, 40 per cent on an individual or family basis and the rest under an employment base (Aufiero 1999). In Brazil, around 740 HMOs of all sizes provide services to 18.3 million people (de Almeida and Rubo 1999). These firms generated revenues of almost US$4 billion in 1998. In Chile, the first Latin American country to open its public system to private solutions, one quarter of the population (3.8 million) are enrolled in private insurance agencies (Piturro 1999). In Colombia, the private sector already accounts for almost 50 per cent of the total enrolment in mandatory plans (Toro-Bridge 1999).

An increasing amount of these pre-paid plans have been implemented or strengthened through joint ventures between local and foreign managed-care firms. Aetna International has developed health plans with 3.3 million members in seven Latin American countries (Schrader 1999). Recently, it acquired, the largest HMO in Argentina. Cigna International has developed joint ventures with local HMOs in

Argentina, Brazil, Chile, Guatemala, and Mexico. The American International Group has established a partnership in Brazil with Unibanco Seguros in a transaction involving US$460 million (Drucker 1999). In Colombia, American, Brazilian, Chilean, and Spanish managed-care companies are already operating.

In addition to clinical services, managed-care processes such as drug-benefit management, transfer of risks to providers, utilization review, and cost-containment strategies) are also being traded in existing health care systems worldwide. Massachusetts-based InterQual is marketing updated clinical protocols in the UK (Berlow and Trig 1997). In Germany, a new law that penalizes physicians whose prescribing exceeds a set target was recently established (Azevedo 1996). A similar principle was recently implemented in the Polish system, where hospitals and not funds now carry the burden of over-expenditure (Nicholls 1999). US AID, while exploring the possibility of developing a pre-paid health care delivery system in Uganda helped in the implementation of a plan under managed-care principles, the HealthPartners Uganda Health Co-operative, that is presently covering 24 000 people (Hahn 1999).

Finally, health care reforms all over the world are favouring the expansion of managed care, which is being considered as part of formal national policies. The importance of health care reform in this respect is most evident in countries such as Chile and the Philippines (Hsaio 1994). Chile introduced reforms in the late 1970s, which eventually favoured the provision of health services through private insurance plans, many of which have adopted managed-care principles. In the early 1980s, the Philippines, encouraged by the publicity about the initial success of American HMOs, promoted the development of these organizations as a lower-cost alternative form of financing and delivering health services. More recently, in central Europe, in response to problems of inefficiency and cost explosion, some countries decided to stop financing their health care systems out of the government's general budget and are experimenting with different financing and provision models including managed care.

Opportunities and challenges

The globalization of health care services has effects on equity, efficiency, and quality of health systems. Table 3.1 summarizes the key opportunities and challenges that arise for each of the four basic forms in which services are exchanged.

Export of services

The export of health care services may lead to an increase in the range of services available in recipient countries, as well as improve access in remote areas. It is likely that it will lead to a more efficient delivery of specialized services and also to an improvement in the timelines and the quality of services in the recipient country.

The main challenges that arise with the export of services are to avoid human and financial resources being spent on highly specialized services that are not cost effective. In addition, exports of services imply substantial investments from the exporting country and require the establishment of quality control standards and regulatory mechanisms.

Table 3.1 Main opportunities and challenges arising from international trade of health services (continued)

	Equity		Efficiency		Quality	
	Opportunities	**Challenges**	**Opportunities**	**Challenges**	**Opportunities**	**Challenges**
Movement of providers	• Increase access to care in recipient countries	• Prevent shortage of providers in exporting countries • Ensure that home country needs are met by training received abroad	• Balance the manpower supply in countries with oversupply	• Deal with the reduced return of investment in training for countries exporting providers	• Increase access to of clinical knowledge and procedures • Favour harmonization of certification procedures	• Prevent negative impacts on the quality of care as a result of exporting providers better trained • Avoid permanent migration of health manpower
Commercial presence	• Improve delivery of service	• Avoid the development of 'multitier' system • Prevent internal brain drains	• Improve access to managerial and information technology • Promote competition and, as a result, cost reduction	• Minimize the transfer of unnecessary medical technology	• Improve access clinical technology • Upgrade and expand health infrastructure • Enhance quality through competition	• Assure appropriate certification and accreditation mechanisms

Movement of health care consumers

The cross-border movement of consumers may also increase the access to cheaper, culturally attractive, or better quality health care services. Recipient countries would benefit from the currency generated by these transactions while sending countries would suffer from capital flight. Because many public and private insurance plans are not portable, consumers receiving care in countries other than their own would not be covered by insurance. For example American retirees living in Latin America, most of whom are covered by Medicare, are not reimbursed for health care expenses incurred outside of the USA. The movement of consumers may provide incentives to the recipient countries to improve the quality of their services. Local health systems will have to ensure that the same quality of services is given to local as to foreign patients, thus preventing preferential treatment of foreigners in attempts to attract foreign currency.

Movement of providers

This also has the opportunity to increase access to health services and promote the exchange of information and clinical procedures among health practitioners and institutions. In addition, it may prompt the harmonization of licensing and certification procedures, with positive impacts on quality of care for those countries with poor regulations.

A possible increase in the flight of skilled personnel from developing countries as a result of trade liberalization and greater professional and economic incentives in developed nations should also be anticipated. Even though some portion of the income of these workers gets remitted back to their country of origin, these countries suffer from flight of talent and loss of the benefits generated by resources invested in training individuals who decide to emigrate. The 111 nurses who withdrew from public service in Jamaica in 1990 cost that country US$1.7 million in training and education costs.

Cross-border establishment of facilities

The establishment of facilities and services in other countries may promote investment, especially in developing countries, creating employment, reducing foreign currency flight, increasing access to technology, upgrading the health infrastructure, and improving the competitive capacity, accessibility, quality, and productivity of services in recipient nations. Access by foreign investment to health services, however, may be limited in the short run since many countries still consider health facilities part of their 'national heritage' and not accessible to trans-national corporations (Price *et al.* 1999).

The possible increase in the costs of care and irrational use of technology are risks related to an increasing commercial presence. In view of the dissemination of a technology-dependent medical culture, national agencies and international co-operation networks will have to be developed to evaluate not only the safety and efficacy of technologic innovations but also their cost effectiveness.

The export of managed-care services may be useful in those countries where private health care is financed out of pocket or through indemnity insurance, helping to limit cost explosions and catastrophic expenditures. The development of solid regulatory infrastructures, however, will be required in order to limit its negative impacts on equity. The experiences of Argentina, Chile, and the Philippines show that for-profit insurance plans and managed-care organizations tend to implement mechanisms to avoid the enrolment of the elderly, the chronically ill, and the disabled, sometimes in spite of the opposing and expensive efforts of the regulatory agencies (Hsaio 1995; Stocker *et al.* 1999).

In strictly commercial terms, developing countries willing to profit from the opportunities offered by the globalization of health care services have a competitive advantage in the low cost of health care within their borders and in certain cultural and geographic factors. On the other hand, firms from developed nations have much better access to capital, technology, administrative knowledge, marketing networks, and highly specialized professional medical services in their favour.

The highest priority will be to guarantee the design and implementation of national and international norms and standards to ensure that trade in services is associated with an equitable access to comprehensive, efficient, and high-quality health care.

The role of the World Trade Organization

A significant factor that is likely to influence the globalization of health care is the growing importance of the WTO and the emphasis that it is placing on the service sector. It is therefore important to understand the nature of this major actor.

The WTO came into existence on 1 January 1995 with 76 governments as members. The membership is now 134. The decision to establish the WTO was taken at the Marrakech Ministerial Conference in 1994 after the completion of the General Agreement on Tariffs and Trade (GATT) Uruguay Round (Koivusalo 1995). WTO replaces the GATT administrative structure and is the legal and institutional foundation of the multi-lateral trading system.

Articles II and III of the agreement establishing the WTO set out the following mandate.

The essential functions of the WTO are:

♦ administering and implementing the multi-lateral and pluri-lateral trade agreements which together make up the WTO

♦ acting as a forum for multi-lateral trade negotiations

♦ seeking to resolve trade disputes

♦ overseeing national trade policies

♦ co-operating with other international institutions involved in global economic policy-making.

The set of agreements that make up the WTO are a single legal instrument that governments must agree to accept in its entirety to accede to membership. These agreements have as their core principle the most-favoured nation treatment (MFN).

This clause requires that trade must be undertaken on the basis of non-discrimination between domestically produced goods and imported products and among imports from different foreign suppliers. Transparency in levels of trade barriers is encouraged through the use of customs tariffs rather than non-tariff measures such as technical standards (Koivusalo 1995). The WTO supplants the existing GATT legal system for trade relations. It forms the basis on which countries frame and implement their domestic trade legislation and regulations.

Like all organizations of the United Nations (UN) system, each WTO member has one vote. This is unlike the Bretton Woods institutions in which power is shared according to financial contributions (Koivusalo 1995). Structurally, the WTO is governed by a Ministerial Conference, which meets at least every two years. This body has the authority to decide on all matters under any of the multi-lateral trade agreements. Members prefer to reach decisions by consensus, not by voting. The General Council oversees the day-to-day operations of the organization and other committees, which handle day-to-day matters related to the different agreements.

Although there is one vote per member, this does not translate into equal power and influence. The WTO is a forum for governments, who are the only ones that can bring forward issues for dispute settlement. The key decisions, however, are made in the advisory bodies to these committees, which are heavily influenced by trans-national corporations. Price and colleagues (Price *et al.* 1999) suggest that 'the trans-national corporations that sit on all important advisory committees decide detailed policy and set the agenda.'

The actual and perceived imbalance between developed and developing countries will have an impact on trade liberalization and on the expected distribution of benefits from the growth in trade.

The World Trade Organization and health

Trade and public health should not be discussed in isolation. Decisions made outside the health sector have a large influence on health outcomes especially for the poor. This was a message of the WHO in a press release (WHO 1999*a*). The WHO also stated that it supports the main purpose of promoting trade, that is, to improve living conditions and to raise real income. Five areas were outlined by the WHO as warranting special attention at the WTO Ministerial Conference in 1999. They are the International Health Regulations, food safety, pharmaceuticals and vaccines, trade in health services, and trade in tobacco products. Specific WTO provisions affect each of these public health areas.

Of particular concern with regard to the International Health Regulations is potential for conflict between this binding international regulatory tool and the WTO Agreement on the Application of Sanitary and Phytosanitary Measures (SPS), as discussed in Chapter 6. This agreement seeks to harmonize national measures for the protection of human, animal, and plant health. While countries retain the right to maintain their own standards, these should not be more restrictive than necessary, and the basic principle of most-favoured nation applies. The agreement stipulates that the international references in matters of food safety are those established by the Codex Alimentarius Commission. The WHO and the Food and Agricultural

Organization of the UN have worked together for many years on the guidelines and recommendations of the Codex Alimentarius Commission. The WHO advocates that decisions made in this area must be science based.

With regard to trade-related aspects of intellectual property rights (TRIPS), WHO supports the incorporation of patent protection into national legislation as stipulated in the agreement. The organization is of the opinion that patents provide an incentive for research and development of new drugs and vaccines and contribute to technological development and to the dissemination of knowledge. The WHO is, however, concerned that access to essential drugs should be safeguarded. This was expressed in a 1999 World Health Assembly resolution, which urged member states to 'explore and review their options under international agreements, including trade agreements, to safeguard access to essential drugs.' In keeping with this the WHO supports the rapid production of generic products, drug prices that are consistent with local purchasing power, and the application of compulsory licensing (as set out in TRIPS) if pricing is abusive or in a national emergency.

The other area in which the WTO has the potential of having a significant impact on the health sector is that of trade in health services. The modes of trade in health services have been discussed earlier in this chapter. The General Agreement on Trade in Services (GATS) is the first multi-lateral agreement to provide a framework for regulating trade in services according to the principles similar to those of trade in other goods. In terms of GATS, health services include the general and specialized services of medical doctors, deliveries and related services, nursing services, physiotherapeutic and paramedical services, all hospital services, ambulance services, residential health facilities services, and services provided by medical and dental laboratories (UNCTAD 1998).

Conclusions

The world enters the twenty-first century with a legacy of changes that will continue to shape the future. The last half century has witnessed what Hobsbawm has described as '. . .the extraordinary scale and impact of economic, social and cultural transformation, the greatest, most rapid and most fundamental in world history' (Hobsbawm 1994). Although complex and contradictory these changes point in the direction of an increased integration among countries.

Globalization *per se* is not a new phenomenon. From time immemorial the forces of trade, migration, war, and conquest have bound together persons from distant places. What is new is the pace and intensity of integration, leading in Hobsbawm's words, to a revolution that has 'virtually annihilated time and distance' (Hobsbawm 1994).

There are potential benefits to trade liberalization in health services. However, as mentioned earlier there is concern that poorer countries may not have a strong enough regulatory framework to ensure that trade issues do not distort their national health priorities (Adams and Kinnon 1998). When framing policy, governments will have to analyse the opportunities and challenges posed by trade liberalization.

Balancing the multiple trade-offs summarized in Table 3.1 will no doubt require enlightened and participatory processes of decision making, both at national and global levels.

Like all other domains of social interaction, health care will be affected profoundly by the greater proximity of people and the goods and services that they produce and trade. The biggest challenge for the policy makers of today is to realize the potential benefits of global integration while safeguarding against new forms of social exclusion and preserving the richness of diversity.

References

Abel-Smith, B. (1986) The world economic crisis: health manpower out of balance. *Health Policy and Planning,* **1**(4), 309–16.

Adams, O. and Kinnon, C. (1998) A public health perspective. In *International trade in health services: a development perspective,* ed. S. Zarilli and C. Kinnin. WHO, Geneva.

Amyes, S. G. B. (2000) The rise in bacterial resistance. *British Medical Journal,* **320,** 199–200.

Aufiero, J. F. (1999) El sistema de salud en la Republica Argentina: propuesta para el sistema nacional de salud. *Fourth Annual Summit on International Managed Care Trends.* December 5–8, Miami, USA.

Azevedo, D. (1996) America's latest export: managed care. *Medical Economics,* December 9, 71–9.

Berlow, B. and Trig, D. (1997) The coming globalization of health care. *Physician Executive,* 23(6), 24–7.

Boufford, J. I. (1995) Potential lessons from the European experience for the North American region. In *Health systems in an era of globalization. challenges and opportunities for North America,* ed. P. Freeman, O. Gomez-Dantes, and J. Frenk. Institute of Medicine (USA)/ National Academy of Medicine (Mexico), Mexico City.

Carlino, M. (1994) Outpatient care: US companies respond to Mexican demand for quality health care. *El Financiero Internacional,* July 25–31, 10–11.

Chen, L., Bell, D., and Bates, L. (1996) World health and institutional change. In *Pocantico retreat. enhancing the performance of international health institutions,* pp. 29–39. The Rockefeller Foundation, Social Science Research Council, Harvard School of Public Health, Cambridge MA.

Chen, L., Evans, T., and Cash, R. (1999) Health as a global public good. In *Global public goods. international cooperation in the 21st century,* ed. I. Kaul, I. Grunberg, and M. Stern, pp. 284–304. Oxford University Press, New York.

de Almeida, A. and Rubo, I. (1999) Health Reform: the private health sector and market opportunities in Brazil. *Fourth Annual Summit on International Managed Care Trends.* December 5–8, Miami, USA.

Desker, B. (1991) Singapore and the provision of medical services for the region. *Singapore Medical Journal,* **32,** 338–90.

Drucker, P. (1999) Beyond the information revolution. *The Atlantic Monthly,* **284**(4), 47–57.

Forum on the Future of Academic Medicine, The physician workforce. http://www.aa.mc.org/about/progemph/forum/issues.htm.

Frenk, J. and Gomez-Dantes, O. (1995) Global integration and health. In *Health systems in an era of globalization. challenges and opportunities for North America*, ed. P. Freeman, O. Gomez-Dantes, and J. Frenk, pp. 62–7. Institute of Medicine (USA)/National Academy of Medicine (Mexico), Mexico City.

Frenk, J., Sepulveda, J., Gomez-Dantes, O. *et al.* (1997) The new world order and international health. *British Medical Journal*, **314**(7091), 1404–7.

Gomez-Dantes, O. and Frenk, J. (1995) NAFTA and health services (initial data). In *Health systems in an era of globalization. challenges and opportunities for North America*, ed. P. Freeman, O. Gomez-Dantes, and J. Frenk, pp. 62–7. Institute of Medicine (USA)/National Academy of Medicine (Mexico), Mexico City.

Gomez-Dantes, O., Frenk, J., and Cruz, C. (1997) Commerce in health services in North America within the context of the North American Free Trade Agreement. *Pan American Journal of Public Health*, **1**(6), 460–5.

Hahn, S. (1999) Health partners Uganda health cooperative serves as new model for health plans in developing countries. *City Business*, December 20.

Hobsbawm, E. (1994) *The age of extremes: a history of the world 1914–1991*. Pantheon Books, New York.

Hsaio, W. C. (1994) Marketization – the illusory magic pill. *Health Economics*, **3**, 351–357.

Hsaio, W. C. (1995) Abnormal economics in the health sector. *Health Policies*, **32**, 125–139.

International Labour Office (1994) The work of strangers: a survey of international labour migration. ILO, Geneva.

Koivusalo, M. (1995) World Trade Organisation and trade-creep in health and social policies. In *Health Economics. WTO: What's In It for WHO?* ed. C. M. Kinnon. WHO Task Force on Health Economics, Geneva

Lagnado, L. (1996) US hospitals target patients from around the Globe. *Wall Street Journal*, August 10, 1.

Larkin, M. (1997) Telemedicine finds its place in the real world. *Lancet*, **350**, 646.

Leidel, R. (1993) Health services and the single market. EC health care systems entering the single market. In *Europe without frontiers. The implications for health*, ed. C. Normand and J. P. Vaughan, pp. 111–18. John Wiley, Chichester.

Medici, A. C., Londono, J. L., Coelho, O. *et al.* 1997) Managed care and managed competition in Latin America and the Caribbean. In *Innovation in health care financing*. World Bank, Washington DC.

McKee M., Mossialos E., Belcher P. (1996) The impact of European Law on national health policy. *Journal of European Social Policy*, **6**, 263–86.

Nicholls, A. (1999) Health and wealth. *Business Central Europe*, **6**(62), 12–17.

OECD (1992) *Services on international transactions 1970–1991*. OECD, Paris.

OECD (1994) *Foreign trade by commodities*. OECD, Paris.

Piturro, M. (1999) Prospect south of the border. Central and Latin America offer new markets and challenges. *Managed Health Care News*, **15**(9), 21–3.

Price, D., Pollock, A., and Shaoul, J. (1999) How the world trade organisation is shaping domestic policies in health care. *Lancet*, **354**, 1889–92.

Schieber, G. and Maeda, A. (1999) Health care financing and delivery in developing countries. *Health Affairs*, May–June.

Schrader, E. (1999) Managed health care latest US export to Mexico (December 5–8). Los Angeles Times, Los Angeles.

Smith, R. (1996) Global competition in health care. *British Medical Journal,* **311**(7060), 764–5.

Stocker, K., Waitzkin, H., and Iriart, C. (1999) The exportation of managed care to Latin America. *New England Journal of Medicine.* **340**(14), 1131–6.

Toro-Bridge, M. (1999) Colombia, private sector and health reforms. *Fourth Annual Summit on International Managed Care Trends.* December 5–8. Miami, USA.

Townsend, R. (1999) Espana duplico en un ano el numero de cigarrillos importados de EEUU. *El Pais,* **11**, 30.

UNCTAD (1998) International trade in health services: difficulties and opportunities for developing countries. In S. Sarrilli and C. Kinnon (eds) *International Trade in Health Services: a Development Perspective,* ed. S. Sarrilli and C. Kinnon. UN/WHO, Geneva.

UNDP (1999) Human development report. UNDP, New York.

Van der Mei, A. P. (1999) The Kohll and Decker rulings: revolution or evolution? *Eurohealth,* **5**(1), 14–15.

Walt, G. (1998) Globalization of international health. *Lancet,* **351**, 434–7.

Waxman, H. S. (1997) Workforce reform, international medical graduates, and the in-training examination. *Annals of Internal Medicine,* **126**(8), 803–4.

Widiatmoke, D. and Gani, A. (1999) International relations within Indonesia's hospital sector. WHO International Regional Conference,Washington DC.

World Bank (1993) *Investing in Health.* Oxford University Press, New York.

WHO (1999*a*) Trade and public health. Why the WHO is at the Third Ministerial Conference of the World Trade Organization. *Third Ministerial Conference of the World Trade Organization.* 30 November–3 December. WHO, Seattle.

WHO (1999*b*) World health report. WHO, Geneva.

WHO (1998) The WHO health statistics. WHO, Geneva.

Chapter 4

Responding to the global challenge of infectious disease

Julius Weinberg

Introduction

The likelihood that an infectious disease outbreak may involve more than one country has been increased by the expansion in international trade and travel. Concern over emerging and re-emerging infectious disease, and the realization that the threat from infectious disease is global has stimulated the development of international collaborations in communicable disease surveillance and response. Communicable disease surveillance and prevention activities should be appropriate for the population at risk, globalization means that this population may now be international.

This chapter will review the development of international responses to the challenges posed by infectious disease and will examine the structures in place today. It will focus in particular on one regional grouping, the European single market, which, with its freedom of movement of goods and labour is an exemplar of the process of globalization. This has brought both threats and the organizational structures to develop responses. The increased awareness of the possibility of outbreaks of communicable disease involving more than one country, and the necessity to co-ordinate investigation of such events has stimulated discussion of the most appropriate mechanism(s) for facilitating and developing communicable disease surveillance at the European level; surveillance has had to follow the market place.

Background

Effective international co-operation in the control of communicable disease has required both advances in scientific knowledge and the willingness of national authorities to co-ordinate action. Although it has long been understood that infectious diseases cross international boundaries, and that communicable disease outbreaks elsewhere are of interest, the establishment of systems for international surveillance of infection is comparatively recent. Infectious disease outbreaks which involve several countries are being recognized increasingly commonly, examples include the following.

+ cholera, trade, and travel (Colwell 1996)

+ shigella (Frost *et al.* 1995) and protozoa (Nichols 2000) contaminating fresh food

- salmonella contaminating packaged food (Killalea *et al.* 1996; Shohat *et al.* 1996)
- meningococcal disease at an international football tournament (Van Loock 1997)
- legionellosis (Ham 1996; Joseph *et al.* 1996) with common exposure to cooling systems.

The nineteenth century

As mentioned in Chapter 1, the present system of international co-operation on infectious disease originated with the first International Sanitary Conference which took place in Paris in 1851 (Howard-Jones 1975). The initial aim was that agreement should be reached on standardized quarantine regulations to prevent the importation of cholera, plague, and yellow fever, seen as posing a threat to Europe. Progress was hampered by lack of understanding of the aetiology or mode of transmission of the diseases under consideration. Indeed, the British delegate did not consider John Snow's (Snow 1849) theory that cholera was transmitted by faecally contaminated water worth a mention. The absence of any firm scientific basis for collaboration meant that the first International Sanitary Conference failed to produce any effective agreement. However it had placed health protection and the notion that nations should interchange information about infectious disease firmly on the international agenda.

The revolution in the understanding of microbiology and the aetiology of communicable disease of the second half of the nineteenth century led to increased recognition of the desirability of establishing mechanisms to prevent the spread of communicable disease. The development of public health nationally was paralleled by awareness of international aspects of communicable disease control; this was driven primarily by concerns over the threat of cholera from Asia. At the fifth International Sanitary Conference held in 1881 a proposal was made to create a permanent International Sanitary Agency of Notification. This was never created because of a lack of support from the participating governments. However an International Sanitary Bureau, later to become the Pan American Sanitary Bureau was established in Washington in 1896 and the Office International d'Hygeine Publique (OIHP) established in Paris in 1907. The OIHP considered the development of standards both for biological products and for the reporting of health statistics as amongst its concerns, presaging the work of the World Health Organization (WHO).

Throughout this period it was not only a lack of scientific knowledge that hampered progress. A central issue that remains important is the tension between disease control and trade (Anonymous 1999)

Between the wars

The notion that disease was a proper subject for international co-operation was strengthened by the Covenant of the League of Nations, which established that members would 'endeavour to take steps in matters of international concern for the prevention and control of disease' (Anonymous 1919). The decision of the USA not to join the League of Nations precluded the development of a single worldwide health organization and three organizations, the Pan American Sanitary Organization, the existing OIHP in Paris and a new Health Committee of the League co-existed.

The World Health Organization

The United Nations conference in 1945 decided upon the establishment of a single organization which would replace the OIHP and the health organization of the League. From the beginning the WHO considered communicable disease surveillance amongst its areas of competence. The influenza epidemic of 1947 stimulated the development of international co-operation between laboratories and competent national authorities leading to the development of national and international reference laboratories for influenza (Goodman 1971). This model was used in the development of a network of WHO collaborating centres.

Under the auspices of the WHO a number of major programmes which required international collaboration between countries and institutions developed. Some of these, such as the eradication of smallpox were spectacularly successful. Many of the collaborations developed were based upon centres of microbiological and virological expertise with a focus on in the establishment of standards for biological reagents, test materials, and procedures. Developments in surveillance tended to lag behind developments in laboratory skills. Whilst international surveillance teams assisted in the investigation of particular problems, longer term surveillance structures, with the regular interchange of data about communicable disease between those with responsibilities in surveillance and control were not developed. Reporting to the WHO for publication in the Weekly Epidemiological Record was a useful exercise for analysis of long-term trends, but not for public health action.

The WHO has also been responsible for administering the International Health Regulations (IHR). The IHR are binding on WHO member states and address cholera, plague, yellow fever, and previously smallpox. Their purpose is to 'ensure the maximum security against the international spread of diseases with a minimum interference with world traffic'. There is considerable anxiety that the IHR have failed to achieve their stated aims. The surveillance infrastructure in not in place in many countries to identify problems, measures that may be taken are perceived as being excessive and there is widespread lack of compliance. The IHR are currently under revision (Anonymous 1999), the aim being to enhance the timeliness of reporting. One idea under consideration is the introduction of 'syndromic reporting', where cases would be notified on the basis of a clinical syndrome, rather than a precise laboratory diagnosis. This would speed up reporting and overcome some of the problems created by the emergence of new infectious agents. This might remove some of the anxieties countries have about the potential economic consequences of reporting certain diseases. New reporting mechanisms will also have to take account of the media, as reports of outbreaks of disease increasingly appear in the press before they have been officially notified.

Current developments

At national level

Increasing problems with communicable disease, in particular the spread of antibiotic resistance and emergence of infections such as legionellosis and the viral haemorrhagic fevers, led to a reawakening of interest in the skills of communicable disease epidemiology and surveillance. In many countries national authorities have responded, often following particularly serious outbreaks, by establishing national centres to co-ordinate and lead communicable disease surveillance.

This development has provided national points of contact and national concentrations of expertise which have facilitated the development of international collaborations in communicable disease and response. However in many parts of the world the infrastructure for communicable disease surveillance at national level is poor. Effective international surveillance collaborations to respond to increasing trade and travel can only be based on good surveillance at national and local levels. Recognition that it is in the interest of wealthy countries to support the development of surveillance at national level in less developed countries may help ensure that the capacity for outbreak recognition is more widely available in the future (Howson *et al.* 1998).

Europe

The development of the European Union (EU), a group of countries within which there is free movement of goods (including foodstuffs), services, and people, has led to a dramatic increase in mobility and has raised the potential for outbreaks of communicable disease which transcend national boundaries. The EU also faces challenges arising from the partial breakdown of public health systems in central and eastern Europe and north Africa that emphasize the vulnerability of populations to events occurring beyond national boundaries, as illustrated by the resurgence of diphtheria in the states of the former USSR and cholera outbreaks in countries bordering the Black Sea, the Caspian Sea, and the Mediterranean.

Further afield, increasing tourism and business travel means that outbreaks of disease have the potential to spread worldwide and no country, region, or community can view itself in isolation. Events such as the outbreak of plague in India (Anonymous 1994) and haemorrhagic fever in the then Zaire (Anonymous 1995) showed the need for national surveillance organizations to react appropriately to events arising far away. This poses a particular challenge to the EU as freedom to move unhindered between states makes harmonization of the member states' response essential. It would be inappropriate for one country to ban flights from an affected area if travellers could fly to a neighbouring country and then cross the border on a train.

The continuing development of the EU has led to the establishment of structures intended to facilitate measures designed to operate at European level. These were strengthened by the signing of the Maastricht Treaty. Article 129 of the treaty provides an explicit basis for EU action in the field of public health: 'the community shall contribute towards ensuring a high level of human health protection by encouraging cooperation between the member states, and if necessary, lending support to their action'. This was developed in Article 152 of the 1997 Amsterdam Treaty, which required that 'a high level of human health protection shall be ensured in the definition and implementation of all Community Policies and activities' (EU 1997).

Whereas national funding bodies tend to be interested in problems apparent at national level, EU institutions are particularly interested in projects which can demonstrate added value from co-operation at European level. This has enabled the establishment of models for international collaboration in communicable disease surveillance which may well be generalizable to other parts of the globe, or which may play a part as the European component of wider international communicable disease collaborations.

USA

The USA, through the Centers for Disease Control (CDC) and the Institute of Medicine have been active in raising the profile of emerging infection and the need for greater international collaboration. This has been exemplified by the production of authoritative reports (Institute of Medicine 1992; Working Group on Emerging and Re-emerging Infectious Diseases 1995) and the development of a new journal *Emerging Infectious Disease*. The CDC has a long tradition of undertaking field epidemiological studies and of supporting training in communicable disease epidemiology in other countries.

The CDC plan for combating infectious disease (Centres for Disease Control and Prevention 1998) makes explicit the importance attached to global issues. Amongst the objectives identified are to:

◆ strengthen global capacity to monitor and respond to emerging infectious diseases

◆ enhance the nation's capacity to respond to complex infectious disease threats in the USA and internationally, including outbreaks that may result from bioterrorism

◆ provide training opportunities in infectious disease epidemiology and diagnosis in the USA and throughout the world

◆ support and promote disease control and prevention internationally.

The World Health Organization

The raised awareness of the problem of 'emerging infectious disease' (Plaut *et al.* 1996) has prompted the development of better international links in communicable disease surveillance in many parts of the world. The WHO has seen a need to strengthen communicable disease surveillance not just at national level, but also internationally, particularly through using information technology (Vacalis *et al.* 1995) developing electronic rapid alert systems, so as to ensure a high level of awareness and preparedness amongst communicable disease epidemiologists.

Within the WHO a Division of Communicable Disease Surveillance and Response has been established. This has enhanced the ability of WHO to undertake epidemiological investigations in the field. The division has published recommendations on surveillance standards which will help in the harmonization of surveillance activities (Department of Communicable Disease Surveillance and Response 1999).

International communicable disease networks

The opening of international borders within the EU within a well-developed legal framework for collaboration has led to the creation of a series of initiatives that offer possible models for other parts of the world. These will now be examined in more detail as they illustrate some of the challenges involved in international collaboration as well as the scope for concerted action. While there is no room for complacency, they have had some success in detecting outbreaks of disease affecting more than one country, in initiating action to reduce the impact of the outbreak upon the population, and in promoting proactive measures to reduce the risks of future events; examples include responses to outbreaks of legionellosis (Joseph *et al.* 1996), shigellosis (Frost *et al.* 1995), and salmonellosis (Killalea *et al.* 1996).

European Working Group on Legionella Infection

A European reporting scheme for travel associated Legionnaires disease was started in 1987 by the European Working Group on Legionella Infection (EWGLI). Twenty-six collaborators in 23 countries have been recruited into the surveillance scheme. The scheme has shown its value in the detection of travel-associated outbreaks of Legionnaires disease which would not have been recognized otherwise (Joseph *et al.* 1996). It has also promoted the establishment of common case definitions and methodologies; and the collaboration of microbiologists and epidemiologists in the investigation of international outbreaks.

A single case of legionella in a returning tourist may not be recognized as belonging to a point source outbreak through national surveillance. The EWGLI database of travel-related legionellosis allows recognition of the fact that patients presenting in several different countries have all had a common exposure.

EnterNet

EnterNet, previously known as Salm-Net, a laboratory-based international human salmonella surveillance collaboration, was established in 1994. The network has already proved effective for the rapid exchange of information concerning international outbreaks of salmonellosis (Killalea *et al.* 1996; Shohat *et al.* 1996), and other enteric organisms (Desenclos *et al.* 1999; Pebody *et al.* 1999). The network has also promoted the development of uniform European typing schemes, and a European data set, so as to enhance the potential for collaborative and comparative work across Europe. Standardized operating procedures have been developed in order to ensure uniformity of procedures between countries in handling information on outbreaks; this is particularly important in establishing safeguards for confidentiality.

The existence, resulting from the establishment of the network, of a group of experts at national level with responsibilities in outbreak investigation has led to the rapid investigation of a number of significant events. 'EnterNet represents an example of how international surveillance systems can be developed to meet the demands of the modern world well into the 21st Century' (EnterNet, website). The EnterNet collaboration has allowed rapid epidemiological assessments of risk to be undertaken following a number of events attributed to internationally traded foodstuffs including infant feed, children's snacks, and salads.

European Antimicrobial Resistance Surveillance System

The international transmission of resistant bacteria has been well documented. This has led to a number of initiatives within the EU including a meeting sponsored by Ministers of Health and the establishment of European Antimicrobial Resistance Surveillance System (EARSS).

The EARSS will co-ordinate the testing of selected micro-organisms in a number of European countries for evidence of anti-microbial resistance using common methods. This will enable better understanding of the problem of anti-microbial resistance at national and at EU level.

Infrastructure developments

Further collaborations have been established which are developing the infrastructure for effective international collaboration. These include:

♦ the European Programme for Intervention Epidemiology Training (EPIET) which involves communicable disease epidemiologists from one country spending two years training in another EU member country, thus developing a body of experts who have experience of working in other systems

♦ early warning systems, rapid alert systems, and access to international data sets (Weinberg *et al.* 1997) being developed under the auspices of the Commission Information and Data for Administrations (IDA) programmes

♦ on-line and published journals for the dissemination of material concerning the surveillance and control of communicable disease (EuroSurveillance Board, website).

Other collaborations are developing around methodologies and other areas of interest to the surveillance community. A study in the EU and its neighbours of national infectious disease surveillance systems (Desenclos *et al.* 1993) concluded that they vary widely in nature, design, and quality and revealed the need for an active, co-ordinated approach to further develop surveillance at the European level. Another study, drawing on lessons from five case studies of different types of outbreaks, made a series of recommendations for enhanced co-operation in the management of outbreaks that involved more than one member state (Brand *et al.* 1999).

Recent developments

There has been considerable debate about how to develop surveillance collaborations, in particular about whether to develop networks or a supra-national centre (Tibayrenc 1997; Bradbury 1998; Editorial 1998; Giesecke and Weinberg 1998). A decision to adopt the network model was taken in September 1998 (European Parliament and Council) and reinforced in November 1998 (European Council of Ministers 1998). This establishes a formal committee of experts who will oversee the development of further networks. This committee will continue the co-ordinating role which had been taken on informally by the 'Charter Group', a committee of the heads of organizations with responsibilities in communicable disease surveillance at national level in the countries of the EU.

The network decision sees the development of a permanent co-ordination structure for communicable disease surveillance in Europe. Although the roles are not completely clear, those presaged by the Charter Group, and which would be relevant to most international collaborations include:

- contributing to the identification of priorities in communicable disease surveillance
- reviewing gaps in European collaborations in communicable disease
- providing advice and helping to establish mechanisms for the interchange of information concerning emerging infections
- helping to develop effective collaborations concerning the surveillance of outbreaks with international implications
- promoting the independent audit and scientific review of collaborations in communicable disease surveillance
- providing advice on scientific standards to collaborations and funding agencies
- developing links with organizations responsible for communicable disease surveillance at national and international level outside the community
- facilitating the development of evidence-based policy.

A number of these actions have already been undertaken. A Delphi study of future priorities for European Collaborations has been published (Weinberg *et al.* 1999) and an inventory of European capacity in communicable disease investigation and control is available from the European Commission on CD-ROM. This will be made available on the Internet in the future.

Information exchange

Information technology and access to the Internet has provided the means for information about outbreaks of infection to be transmitted rapidly and widely. This clearly has benefits, as alerts can be made more timely. However there are also drawbacks. Unsubstantiated rumours may be transmitted and may require extensive investigation to confirm or refute.

Internet-based information exchange systems range from the informal such as ProMED, an open e-mail list with 40 000 subscribers worldwide (ProMED, website; Mitchell, P. 1997), to closed rapid alert systems between surveillance systems. Rapid information exchange proved invaluable when an alert about a single case of an unusual septicaemia in a drug addict prompted recognition that this was a problem that had affected more than one country, and was a consequence of the international trade in narcotics.

The rapid transmission of information is being accompanied by the development of systems for the validation of information being led by the WHO.

The future of global collaborations

It is likely that the international dimension of communicable disease will remain an area of growing activity. International collaboration will become increasingly important in the acute phase of an event to allow early warning and appropriate response. There are now several examples of how the growth in understanding of the relationship between disease and factors such as climate can be used to predict at least the conditions that make outbreaks likely if not the outbreaks themselves (Mitchell, P. 1997; Epstein 1999; Linthicum *et al.* 1999).

In the longer term collaborations are essential to develop the infrastructure for surveillance at national and local level and to ensure that harmonization of methods occurs. Not all countries will be able to afford to undertake all the investigations necessary. Laboratory support has often been provided by CDC, the WHO collaborating centres, or the network of Institut Pasteur laboratories. International inventories of communicable disease resources are being developed so that appropriate support facilities can be identified rapidly.

The model provided by the EU may not be appropriate to all parts of the world, however it appears likely that other regional networks, linking areas with common epidemiological problems will develop. The major challenge lies in ensuring the funding of regional networks and the development of national surveillance in resource-poor areas.

The most important developments are likely to be:

♦ improved information links, with the development of improved, validated rapid alert systems, and consistent international data sets

♦ harmonization of case definitions and surveillance methodology

♦ harmonization of laboratory methods and identification schemes.

Experience developing international networks in communicable disease has shown that they are effective in detecting and informing the control of communicable disease threats. The strength of collaborations lies within the network of networks that has developed, bringing experts together regularly, developing common systems and approaches with the development of common case definitions for surveillance, and harmonizing the epidemiological and microbiological methods and standards and training in communicable disease surveillance. There is inevitably potential for misunderstanding and mistakes which systems need to be able to withstand. Networks need to be based on sound principles and be subject to regular external scientific review. The need for effective international surveillance of infectious disease will continue. A number of models may well develop to serve the needs of different parts of the world. However underlying all of these will be a requirement to build an international body of experts with a variety of overlapping areas of interest and skill, who share common approaches and, most importantly trust one another.

The contribution of the health professional

So far, this chapter has focused on international structures that have been developed in response to the international and global threat from communicable diseases. In general, they are based on agreements between governments and with international agencies. As such, they might seem rather remote from the concerns of individual health professionals. This is, however, wrong. Many were created initially by groups of pioneering individuals, only later to be brought into the mainstream of international structures. Some, such as EWGLI, continue to depend on large amounts of goodwill and short-term project funding. The practical implementation of international responses to communicable disease, at least in Europe, has thus been driven by individual health professionals rather than governments.

Their efforts can be successful only if they buld upon the activities of many other health professionals, most of whom will be unaware of the key role that they can play.

However effective the international mechanisms put in place are, the control of infectious disease depends upon the actions taken at the point where the threat to health is first recognized. Effective control depends upon health professionals and others recognizing the problem as early as possible and reporting it rapidly to those with a responsibility for action and a rapid response. In many countries the reporting of communicable disease remains inadequate and the response is delayed. Many health professionals remain unaware of their responsibility to inform public health authorities, and those authorities are often inadequately staffed and poorly resourced.

Improving national infrastructures, with greater involvement of health professionals and feedback to them is essential. This must be underpinned by improved laboratory support and the appropriate use of information technology. The move towards syndromic reporting may improve the reporting of events.

Infectious disease control relies upon the integration of clinical, epidemiological, and laboratory skills. Health professionals with each of these sets of skills need to recognize their responsibilities and their interdependence if the goal of reducing the international threat to health from infectious disease is to be achieved.

References

Altman, D. (1999) Globalisation political economy, and HIV/AIDS. *Theory and Society,* **28,** 559–84.

Anonymous (1919) Article XXIII Covenant of the League of Nations. Geneva.

Anonymous (1994) Plague. India. *Weekly Epidemiological Record,* **69**(39), 289–91.

Anonymous (1995) Ebola haemorrhagic fever. *Weekly Epidemiological Record,* **70**(34), 241–2.

Bradbury, J. (1998) European infectious diseases centre takes shape. *Lancet,* **352,** 969.

Brand, H., Camaroni, I., Gill, N. *et al.* (1999) An evaluation of the arrangements for managing an epidemiological emergency involving more than one EU member state. Institute of Public health, NRW, Bielefeld.

Centres for Disease Control and Prevention (1998) Preventing emerging infectious diseases. A strategy for the 21st century. CDC Atlanta, Georgia.

Colwell, R. (1996) Global climate and infectious disease: the cholera paradigm. *Science,* **274,** 2025.

Department of Communicable Disease Surveillance and Response (1999) WHO recommended surveillance standards, 2nd edn. WHO, Geneva.

Desenclos, J., Fisher, I., and Gill, N. (1999) Management of the investigation by Enter-net of international foodborne outbreaks of gastrointestingal organisms. *Eurosurveillance,* **4,** 58–62.

Desenclos, J. C., Bijkerk, H., and Huisman, J. (1993)Variations in national infectious diseases surveillance in Europe. *The Lancet*, 1003–6.

Editorial (1998) Not another European Institution. *Lancet*, **352**, 1237.

EnterNet Home of the international surveillance network for the enteric infections – Salmonella and VTEC 0157, http://www2.phls.co.uk.

Epstein, P. R. (1999) Climate and health (comment). *Science*, **285**(5246), 347–8.

EU (1997) Treaty of Amsterdam. EU, Brussels.

European Council of Ministers (1998) Council Conclusions of 26 November 1998 on the future framework for Community action in the field of public health. EU, Brussels.

European Parliament and Council Decision No 2119/98/EC of the European Parliament and of the Council of 24 September 1998 setting up a network for the epidemiological surveillance and control of communicable diseases in the community. EU, Brussels.

EuroSurveillance Board Eurosurveillance, http://www.eurosurv.org.

Frost, J., McEvoy, M., Bently, C. *et al.* (1995) An outbreak of Shigella sonnei infection associated with consumption of iceberg lettuce. *Emerging Infectious Disease*, **1**, 26–9.

Giesecke, J. and Weinberg, J. (1998) A European centre for infectious disease? *Lancet*, **352**, 1308.

Goodman, N. (1971) *International health organizations and their work*. Churchill Livingstone, Edinburgh.

Ham, C. (1996) Population-centred and patient-focused purchasing: the UK experience. *Milbank Quarterly*, **74**(2), 191–214.

Howard-Jones, N. (1975) The scientific background of the international sanitary conferences 1851–1938. WHO, Geneva.

Howson, C., Fineberg, H., and Bloom, B. (1998) The pursuit of global health: the relevance of engagement for developed countries. *The Lancet*, **351**, 586–90.

Institute of Medicine (1992) *Emerging infections: microbial threats to health in the United States*. National Academy Press, Washington, DC.

Joseph, C., Morgan, D., and Birtles, R. (1996) An international investigation of an outbreak of legionnaires disease among UK and French tourists. *European Journal of Epidemiology*, 1–5.

Killalea, D., Ward, L., Roberts, D. *et al.* (1996) International epidemiological and microbiological study of an outbreak of *Salmonella agona* infection from a ready to eat savoury snack 1: England and Wales and the United States. *British Medical Journal*, **313**, 1105–7.

Linthicum, K. J., Anyamba, A., Tucker, C. J. *et al.* (1999) Climate and satellite indicators to forecast Rift Valley fever epidemics in Kenya. *Science*, **285**(5246), 397–400.

Nichols, G. L. (2000) Food-borne protozoa. *British Medical Bulletin*, **56**(1), 209–35.

Pebody, R., Furtado, C., Rojas, A. *et al.* (1999) An international outbreak of Vero cytotoxin-producing Escherichia coli 0157 infection amongst tourists; a challenge for the European infectious disease surveillance network. *Epidemiology and Infection*, **123**, 217–23.

Plaut, M., Hughes, J., and Berkelman, R. (1996) A global theme issue on emerging and re-emerging global microbial threats. *Journal of the American Medical Association*, **27**(6), 197–8.

ProMED http://www.promedmail.org.

ProMED-mail Mitchell, P. (1997) Outbreak intelligence or rash reporting? *Lancet*, **350**, 1610.

Public Health and Trade Anonymous (1999) Revision of the International Health Regulations. Comparing the roles of 3 international organizations. *WER*, **25**, 193–201.

Revision of the IHR Anonymous (1999) Progress report. *WER*, **30**, 252–3.

Shohat, T., Green, M., Merom, D. *et al.* (1996) International epidemiological and microbiological study of an outbreak of Salmonella agona infection from a ready to eat savoury snack –2: Israel. *British Medical Journal*, **313**,1107–9.

Snow, J. (1849) *On the mode of communication of cholera.* Churchill, London.

Tibayrenc, M. (1997) European centres for disease control. *Nature*, **389**, 433.

Vacalis, T., Barlettt, C., and Shapiro, C. (1995) Electronic communication and the future of international public health surveillance. *Emerging Infectious Disease*, **1**(1), 34–5.

Van Loock, F. (1997) Meningococcal disease associated with an international youth football tournament in Belgium. *Eurosurveillance Weekly*, **1**, 970619.

Weinberg, J., Nohynek, H., and Giesecke, J. (1997) Development of a European electronic network on communicable diseases: the IDS-HSSCD programme. *Eurosurveillance*, **2**, 51–3.

Weinberg, J., Grimaud, O., and Newton, L. (1999) Establishing priorities for European collaboration in communicable disease surveillance. *European Journal of Public Health*, **9**, 236–40.

Working Group on Emerging and Re-emerging Infectious Diseases (1995) Infectious disease – a global health threat. Committee on International Science, Engineering and Technology (CISET), National Science and Technology Council, Washington DC.

Chapter 5

Climate change and stratospheric ozone depletion

Tony McMichael and Alistair Woodward

Introduction

The scale of human impact on the natural environment has multiplied greatly over the past two centuries, as the number of humans has grown and as the intensity of economic activity has increased (McMichael 1993; Meyer 1996). The earlier symptoms of this impact, such as industrial air pollution and chemical pollution of waterways, are now being supplemented with worldwide changes to some of the planet's great biophysical systems, including the climate system, the stratospheric ozone layer, the hydrological cycle, soil fertility, and biodiversity. We are beginning, unintentionally, to alter the conditions of life on Earth – and we cannot know in advance the full range of consequences.

Epidemiologists have begun to undertake the complex assessment of the health consequences of these global environmental changes. This requires both the expansion of existing knowledge about climate/environment and health relationships and the use of this knowledge to forecast the likely future health impacts of these large-scale environmental changes. The initial approach has been rather reductionist; that is, the assessment of potential health impacts has been conducted for each global change process separately. Nevertheless, attempts are now being made to study, and model, the combined impacts of coexistent global environmental changes.

Multi-disciplinary scientific networking in relation to these global changes began in earnest in the mid-1980s, particularly under the aegis of the United Nations (UN) system. The UN Environment Program (UNEP) assumed responsibility for assessing the risks posed by stratospheric ozone depletion to human health, to other species, and to ecosystem functioning. The UN General Assembly established the Intergovernmental Panel on Climate Change (IPCC) in 1988, under the joint supervision of the World Meteorological Organization and UNEP.

During the 1980s, the international scientific community, through the International Council of Scientific Unions, set up the International Geosphere Biosphere Project (IGBP). The IGBP nurtured and supported a range of interdisciplinary initiatives in the general 'earth sciences' realm. Shortly after, social scientists established the International Human Dimensions (of Global Environmental Change) Project (IHDP). Both IGBP and IHDP have, in recent years, extended their field of vision to consideration of the impacts of large-scale environmental and social-demographic changes upon human population health.

Meanwhile, various non-governmental organizations have paid increasing attention to global environmental change. Greenpeace International, for example, has supplemented its longstanding concerns over local environmental pollution and the endangering of particular species with active research and advocacy in relation to climate change, ozone depletion, biodiversity loss, and other global environmental changes. The WorldWide Fund for Nature (WWF) and the International Union for the Conservation of Nature (IUCN) are playing increasingly prominent roles in relation to these problems, and have undertaken new liaisons with bodies such as the World Bank. These moves reflect a nascent recognition of the risks to future human well-being and health posed by these historically unprecedented global environmental changes.

This emerging awareness of the potential wide-ranging consequences of eroding the biosphere's life-support systems is adding new depth to the policy discourse. There is growing acceptance of the need for unprecedented international collaboration to achieve the necessary sustainability transition – that is, a move to sustainability of ecological systems and an environmental resource base that supports healthy life, not merely the more superficial sustainability of economic indicators, employment, and recreational amenity. We will require some radical reconfiguration of our social and economic structures, values, and practices. Earlier demographic and epidemiological transitions were associated with industrialization, economic growth, social modernization, and increasing consumerism and led to longer-lived and larger populations with increasing material aspirations. The early, self-generating transitions have, in fact, created the conditions of global environmental change that now necessitate a deliberate sustainability transition (McMichael *et al.* 2000*b*).

Because considerations of the sustainability of population health are central to this policy discourse, public health scientists have an important role to play. They are seeking to improve their capacity to forecast the future health consequences of these emergent global environmental changes. The primary challenge for policy makers and the public is to incorporate the idea of ecological sustainability into social structures, economic practice, and technological choice – such that the conditions for good health can be maintained while material standards of living, along with socially supportive environments, can also be upheld.

Global environmental change: the view from the top

In September 1999 the UN Environment Programme issued an important report: *Global Environment Outlook 2000* (UNEP 1998). Its final chapter begins thus:

> The beginning of a new millennium finds the planet Earth poised between two conflicting trends. A wasteful and invasive consumer society, coupled with continued population growth, is threatening to destroy the resources on which human life is based. At the same time, society is locked in a struggle against time to reverse these trends and introduce sustainable practices that will ensure the welfare of future generations . . .

There used to be a long time horizon for undertaking major environmental policy initiatives. Now time for a rational, well-planned transition to a sustainable system is running out fast. In some areas, it has already run out: there is no doubt that it is too late to make an easy transition to sustainability for many of these issues . . .

The report urges national governments to recognize the need for urgent, concerted, and radical action. Notice particularly the emphasis on the word 'sustainability'.

Disappointingly, the report's coverage of the consequent risks to human population health is weak. Its briefly stated environmental health concerns are mostly about toxic chemical pollutants. There is little reference to the ways in which a weakened biosphere with disrupted ecosystems, altered biogeochemical cycling, and depleted natural capital would impinge on human health – via, for example, reduced food yields, fresh water shortages, eutrophication of waterways, altered patterns of infectious disease transmission, and displacement of marginal and unprotected populations.

This particular weakness in the report echoes a corresponding weakness in the 1987 report of the World Commission on Environment and Development – a report that had little to say about human health, other than to note its importance as a resource for economic development (World Commission on Environment and Development 1987). In the World Health Report of 1999, the World Health Organization (WHO) Director-General, Dr Brundtland, welcomed greater collaboration between UN agencies, the World Bank and the International Monetary Fund (IMF) to address health and poverty (WHO 1999). She noted that: 'A five year difference in life expectancy may yield an extra annual growth of 0.5 per cent. It is a powerful boost to economic growth.' This view appears to characterize population health principally as an asset, as a means to an economic end – although later in her commentary Brundtland also stressed that health is a 'fundamental human right'.

This recurring misconnect between environment and health is also a reminder that, repeatedly, around the world, these sectors do not communicate satisfactorily with one another. UNEP should be tackling the issue of environment and health jointly with WHO. We also see this sectoral separateness routinely at the level of national government. For the moment, policy-makers in the environment and health sectors are often pursuing different priorities, seemingly motivated by divergent value systems – and divergent political imperatives. This separateness is paradoxical. After all, a prime reason for seeking to maintain environmental quality is to protect the health of humans and other species – and a prime determinant of population health in the medium-to-long term is the life-supporting capacity of the environment. If we had a clearer understanding of this fundamental *ecological* relationship between environmental conditions and population biology and health, then these sectors would work more closely together.

Human impact on the Earth: our expanding 'ecological footprint'

Because of the great and growing weight of humankind upon the world's environment we have begun to weaken or deplete various natural biophysical systems on a global scale (McMichael 1993; Vitousek *et al.* 1997). The best-known example of human-induced global environmental change is our incipient impact on the climate system because of changes in the energy-absorbing gaseous composition of the lower atmosphere. But that is just one of several large-scale environmental changes. We are continuing to deplete stratospheric ozone; we are extinguishing species and reducing biodiversity; the spread of invasive species (plants, animals, microbes) is increasing; we have changed the global cycling of nitrogen and sulphur; fresh water supplies are coming under pressure; and so are the food-producing ecosystems on land and at sea.

These large-scale environmental changes entail a direct weakening of the bio-sphere's life-supporting infrastructure. This necessarily jeopardizes the *sustainability* of human health. It is important that the enlarged and *ecological* dimension of this problem category be appreciated. In process terms, it is more than a simple extension of the long-standing problem of local environmental pollution and degradation. It takes us into the realm of an impending ecological crisis, because it entails an overloading of the biosphere, exceeding global carrying capacity.

In recent decades the scale of human intervention in the natural world has escalated enormously (Meyer 1996; McMichael and Powles 1999). The 'size' of the global economy has increased approximately 20-fold this century. We are now clearly operating in ecological deficit. Current economic growth, with prevailing technology, now depends substantially on our continued consumption of natural capital. For example, it has been estimated that the cities of the Baltic region require an area of the Earth's surface several hundred times greater than the aggregate area of those cities in order to sustain the supply of material and to absorb the cities' wastes (Folke *et al.* 1996). This ecological deficit is evident in recent published estimates of the decline in global ecosystem indices made by the WWF (Loh *et al.* 1998) and estimates of the current and growing size of humankind's collective 'ecological footprint' (Wackernagel and Rees 1995). Both estimates suggest that humankind currently is significantly dependent on consuming natural capital in order to maintain present production, consumption, and waste absorption levels.

This suggests an important distinction between how we think about 'environmental sustainability' and 'ecological sustainability'. The former tends, by current usage, to refer to maintaining purity of environmental media: air, water, soil, and food. The latter refers to the maintenance of stocks of natural capital, including fully functioning ecosystems and other bio-geochemical systems (such as climate). The former is usually not a true problem of sustainability – London's air can be thick with particulates one decade, and much cleaner in the following decade. That is, the future is not being foreclosed for oncoming generations of inhalers. The violation of ecological sustainability, however, entails an overload of the biosphere's carrying capacity, such that stocks of some natural resources are depleted and some things are lost, or changed, irreversibly – or at least for a very long time. The prospects for future generations are thus diminished.

Before considering how these ideas bear on strategies for co-operative action to arrest the destruction of stratospheric ozone and the excessive emission of greenhouse gases, we should review the likely health consequences of these two global environmental changes.

The potential health impacts of climate change

A change in global climate due to human-induced alteration of atmospheric composition is now widely anticipated by climatologists (Houghton *et al.* 1995). The Second Assessment Report of the UN's IPCC, in 1996, concluded that: 'The balance of evidence suggests a discernible human influence on global climate'.

Changes in world climatic conditions and patterns over the coming century would have wide-ranging consequences for human health (McMichael *et al.* 1996; McMichael and Haines 1997). A change in climate – and, more particularly, in climate variability – would increase the exposure of many populations to extreme weather events. Climate change may also stress the systems and institutions through which public health and nutrition programmes are implemented. By stretching limited social resources across a broader range of health and other problems, a change in climate could thus leave these pubic health programmes under-resourced and therefore less effective.

Climate change would affect human health via paths of varying complexity, scale, and directness. The timing of the various types of impacts would differ. The forecasting of health impacts entails dealing with complex and dynamic processes, multiple uncertainties, a variable time-horizon – and, often, surprises (Levins 1995; McMichael 1997). Many of the health impacts would arise from disturbance or weakening of the biosphere's biophysical systems. Some impacts, in some regions, would be beneficial; most impacts, however, would be adverse. Long-term changes in world climate would affect many of the foundations of public health – sufficient food, safe and adequate drinking water, secure community settlement and family shelter, and the environmental and social control of various infectious diseases.

The more direct impacts include those due to changes in exposure to weather extremes (summer heatwaves, winter cold), those due to increases in other extreme weather events (floods, cyclones, storm-surges, droughts, etc.), and those due to increased production of certain air pollutants and aeroallergens (spores and moulds). In assessing these impacts, there is a general need to consider the balance of beneficial and adverse effects. For example, decreases in winter mortality due to milder winters may compensate for increases in summer mortality due to the increased frequency of heatwaves. In countries with a high level of excess winter mortality, such as the UK, the beneficial impact may outweigh the detrimental (Department of Health 2000). The extent to which the frequency of extreme weather events will be altered by climate change remains uncertain, although many climatologists predict a change in the pattern of floods and droughts. Large-scale migration may occur in response to climate-induced changes in food supply, and to flooding, drought and other natural disasters.

The effects of climate change upon infectious disease transmission would entail essentially indirect mechanisms. The distribution and abundance of vectors and intermediate hosts are determined by various physical factors (temperature, precipitation, humidity, surface water, and wind) and biotic factors (vegetation, host species, predators, competitors, parasites, and human interventions). Various integrated modelling studies have forecast that an increase in ambient temperature would cause, worldwide, net increases in the geographic distribution of particular vector organisms – such as malarial mosquitoes – although some localized decreases may also occur (Focks *et al.* 1995; Martens *et al.* 1999). Further, temperature-related changes in the life-cycle dynamics of both the vector species and the pathogenic organisms (flukes, protozoa, bacteria, and viruses) would increase the potential transmission of many vector-borne diseases such as malaria, dengue, and leishmaniasis.

Climate change may effect the transmission of water-borne infectious diseases via several mechanisms. The primary mechanism will be intensification of the rainfall cycle, leading either to flooding that causes contamination of water supplies, or drought that depletes drinking water supplies. Bacterial water-borne illnesses such as cholera and parasitic diseases such as cryptosporidiosis may thus be affected.

Some recent evidence indicates that global warming alters the atmospheric heat budget so as to increase the cooling of the stratosphere (Shindell *et al.* 1998). If such stratospheric cooling continues, the risk of ozone depletion could continue to increase even after chlorine and bromine loading starts to decline in response to implementation of the (severally amended) Montreal Protocol of 1987.

Collateral health risks: a prospect for win–win solutions?

The pressing needs of the world's present public health problems appear to compete with addressing scenario-based future risks to health. Clearly, we must not neglect the present in order to worry about the future. But do the public health needs of the present really compete with those of the future? In reality, both types of problems have their origins in common underlying fundamentals – as manifested in persistent poverty and inequity, in the promotion of materials-intensive production and consumption, in environmental mismanagement, and in a declining capacity to control many serious infectious disease agents.

There are other types of connections between present and future. Consider the case of health risks in relation to fossil fuel combustion – which releases noxious pollutants into the local air and carbon dioxide into the atmosphere at large. We can estimate the savings that would result from a reduction of fossil fuel combustion, undertaken to mitigate greenhouse gas emissions. For the world as a whole, it has been estimated approximately that seven million premature deaths due to air pollution could be avoided by 2020 if there were worldwide compliance with Kyoto Protocol-level carbon dioxide emission reductions (Working Group on Public Health and Fossil-Fuel Combustion 1997). Related estimations for China indicate that, if that country were to comply with the carbon dioxide emission cutbacks of the Kyoto Protocol, then by 2020 the annual avoidance of premature deaths from ambient (external) air pollution in China would be in the range of 2000–16 000 (Wang and Smith 2000) – while the equivalent number of avoidable deaths for the simultaneous reductions in indoor exposure (where coal is currently the main domestic fuel and exposures are often extreme) would be a vast 50 000 to 500 000. The width of those ranges reflects both the existence of alternative technological approaches to emission reductions and the uncertainties of the dose-specific risks to health.

Stratospheric ozone depletion

Since the mid-1970s scientists have known that stratospheric ozone was being depleted, especially in the later winter and early spring and predominantly at high latitudes, by human-made gases such as chloroflurocarbons (CFCs). Ambient ground-level levels of ultraviolet irradiation are estimated to have increased consequently by up to 10 per cent at mid-to-high latitudes over the past two decades (Slaper et al. 1996). Via the Montreal Protocol of 1987, updated in the 1990s, the release of many of these gases has been curtailed. However, a problem remains with black-market sales and with the escalating production of halons by China and other low-income countries temporarily exempted from the production ban.

For at least the first two-thirds of the twenty-first century, we can expect the ongoing increase in ultraviolet radiation exposure to augment the severity of sunburn, the incidence of skin cancers, and the incidence of various disorders of the eye (especially cataracts). Scenario-based modelling, integrating the processes of emissions accrual in the stratosphere, consequent ozone destruction, increased UVR flux, and cancer induction, indicates that European and US populations will experience a 5–10 per cent excess in skin cancer incidence during the middle decades of the coming century (Slaper et al. 1996). Similar modelled projections have been made for other fair-skinned populations living in Australia and New Zealand (Martens 1998).

Increased ground-level exposure to ultraviolet radiation could also cause some suppression of immune functioning, thus increasing susceptibility to infectious diseases and perhaps reducing vaccination efficacy (UNEP 1998). Another potentially important, though indirect, health detriment could arise from ultraviolet-induced impairment of photosynthesis on land (terrestrial plants) and at sea (phytoplankton), Although such an effect could reduce the world's food production, few data are yet available.

Health impacts of other global environmental changes

World per capita production of cereal grains has plateaued since the mid-1980s. This may indicate that we are approaching the limits of practically achievable per-hectare yields – although there are other contributory explanations (Dyson 1999). There is little potential new arable land available – and much of the land in use has already been badly managed and damaged. The UN's Food and Agricultural Organization (FAO) has documented the difficulties in reducing food insecurity in the world as population pressures and land degradation undermine attempts to boost yields (FAO 1999).

The FAO estimates that ocean fisheries are also at their yield limit (100 million tonnes per year), and it appears that several fisheries – including the once-bountiful Grand Banks (north-west Atlantic) cod fishery – have collapsed or been seriously damaged (FAO 1995). Beyond some anticipated gains from large-scale mariculture and marginal gains from genetic engineering (for example for disease resistance), technical advances equivalent to those that enabled the Green Revolution of the 1960s and 1970s seem unlikely. One reason is that photosynthetic yields from crop plants seem already to have been maximized (Greenland et al. 1998).

Only a brief mention can be made here of the other large-scale environmental changes that characterize today's world, such as fresh water (especially aquifer) depletion, accelerating losses of biodiversity, the spread of invasive species, and rapid urbanization of the human population. These all have potentially serious consequences for human health (McMichael 1993; Watson *et al.* 1998). In particular, many of these processes influence agricultural yields and the pattern of infectious disease transmission.

Causes of population vulnerability to climate change: opportunities for international action

How severely public health is affected by climate change will depend on the magnitude and rate of change, and the degree to which populations can adapt to the new environment. There is a growing interest amongst scientists and policy makers in questions of vulnerability and adaptation (Box 5.1). Of course it remains very important to find ways of reducing future greenhouse emissions, but even if international agreements such as the Kyoto protocols are put into practice carbon dioxide levels will continue to rise for some time yet. Moreover, to a degree climate change is already committed as a result of greenhouse gases emitted in the past. International actions in response to climate change must include both mitigation (controlling the causes of global warming) and adaptation (increasing the capacity of populations to respond to climate change in a positive fashion).

Vulnerability ('the capacity for loss') may be individual or collective. It applies both to resistance to change, and to the ability to recover once changes have occurred. Plainly there are biological and physical causes of vulnerability. For example, large-scale clearances of forests change the physical landscape and increase the likelihood of losses following heavy rainfall since levels of run-off are higher and flows are more rapid. In the same way geography dictates, to a large extent, vulnerability to the effects of sea-level rise. Many populations in the Pacific are on the physical margins of sustainable settlement, and the combined effects of coastal erosion, rising salinity, reduced rainfall, and inundation are serious threats to a number of island states.

However vulnerability is not entirely determined by geography or history. The extent and rate of forest clearances depends on a host of factors including government policies, whether or not these policies are enforced, and conditions of trade. Likewise, patterns of land use in coastal areas will make a large difference to the consequences of sea level rise. Vulnerability has a social dimension and in a practical sense the social dimension is the most important aspect of all, since policies, regulations and the activities of public agencies are often more susceptible to change than factors in the physical environment or biological attributes.

What are the major social causes of vulnerability to disease and injury resulting from climate variability and climate change? To a large extent the important underlying causes are not peculiar to climate change. Impoverished populations are likely to be at greater risk because they have fewer choices than those with resources at their disposal. However poverty and vulnerability are not synonymous. Overconsumption may also increase the likelihood of future losses: for example, rapid increases in population size, density of settlement, and use of natural resources may compromise

Box 5.1: **International action to reduce vulnerability**

The IPCC Special Report on Technology Transfer concluded that there are three components of effective aid. These are 'hardware' (providing the equipment for monitoring, communicating, and responding to environmental threats), human capital (education and training), and social development (building institutions, networks, and public understanding and support for change) (IPCC in press). The third element is often overlooked, but adapting to long-term climate change requires substantial, deep-seated changes, and it is naive to expect that these can be simply achieved by importing machines and technicians. The World Bank drew a similar conclusion recently: 'institutions matter' was one of the four key messages of the 1999/2000 World Development Report, 'sustained development should be rooted in policies that are socially inclusive and responsive to changing circumstances' (World Bank 1997).

It is logical that aid should be focused on the regions, countries, and groups that face the greatest risk of losses due to climate change, and this has spurred the development of measures of vulnerability. A number of new indices have been reported, including measures of vulnerability to environmental damage (Kaly *et al.* 1999), famine (Downing and Bakker 1999), and economic losses (Briguglio 1993). Still needed are techniques and measures to identify places and populations at greatest risk of ill health due to a changing global climate.

Action to reduce vulnerability to changes in the physical environment must take account of the international economic environment since this has a powerful influence on decisions taken nationally. For example, a more open international trading system may lead to a wider distribution of economic benefits, but 'this requires linkage to sound social policies, including the recognition of health as a global public good' (Drager 1999). There must be linkages also to measures that will ensure protection of the environment. Under the present system there are two problems: first, the full costs of economic activity (including those resulting from environmental damage) do not appear on standard balance sheets; and, second, these costs are borne unequally.

In the Pacific (and elsewhere) a history of dependency dating to the colonial period and increasingly adverse terms of trade commonly combine with serious damage to local natural environments. In the Solomon Islands and a number of other countries in the region, for example, logging operations in native forests proceed at a rate that is not sustainable and seriously increases the risks of erosion, slippage, and flooding; yet these operations bring few economic, social, or environmental benefits to local communities (Schep 1997). An important reason why these destructive and maladaptive activities occur is that countries such as the Solomon Islands lack clout at the international negotiating table. The integrity of health-sustaining environments in the Pacific will remain at risk until the world trade system introduces more effective mechanisms to protect the interests of small states.

responsiveness by damaging the buffering capacity of ecological systems. The structure of societies and the ways in which key decisions are made are important. For example, aspects of social 'connectedness' are strongly related to the ability of individuals and populations to recover from natural disasters (Sen 1981). Flexibility and inclusiveness in political decision-making process are also factors that are important in recovery following disasters (Woodward *et al.* 1998). External relations play a part as well. Dependency (such as reliance on others for information and vital goods) carries high risks since it means that essential resources may not be available when they are most needed.

An example of vulnerability and its causes is the threat to food security in the Pacific, a region which contributes each year less than two per cent of the global total of greenhouse gases but stands to lose heavily from rising sea levels and other forecast manifestations of climate change.

Climate change threatens the production, distribution, and storage of food, as a result of long-term processes such as erosion and salination, and acute events including drought, floods, and storms (Parry and Rosenzweig 1993). Traditional communities in the Pacific were familiar with droughts and storms and the threat of hunger. In response they developed strategies for securing food supplies (Pollock 1992). These included the cultivation of staple crops that were relatively storm- and drought-resistant (such as yams and taro), maintaining a diversity of food sources and preserving food using techniques (such as fermentation and drying) that were well suited to island conditions. There were also social buffers against famine. Kin networks within islands meant that food was likely to be shared in times of hardship, and well-established inter-island trading systems provided a wider circle of exchange partners.

It is ironic that 'development' in the region has in some ways increased the vulnerability of Pacific islanders to food shortages. There has been a general move to cash-cropping, often relying on single crops (such as coconuts, banana, or pumpkin). Local food production has fallen away in many places and some communities are dependent on imported staples such as rice, tinned fish, and frozen meat. Traditional methods of food preservation have been replaced by refrigeration, which is effective so long as there is an uninterrupted power supply. Migration, urban drift, and cultural change mean that local social networks are often weaker than in the past and trade links from the islands are chiefly with distant metropolitan states rather than near neighbours (Campbell 1999).

It is important to appreciate that the pattern of change varies widely across the Pacific. For example, in the 1980s levels of food imports ranged from relatively low in Kiribati to very high in Micronesia, with states such as Vanuatu and Tonga in between. Very little home-grown food at all is consumed in French Polynesia, while in the Solomon Islands during the 1980s consumption of fresh fish actually increased at the expense of tinned fish (Cameron 1997). The health effects of these changes in dietary patterns have also been mixed, including benefits (due to greater access to high protein foods and mineral supplements, for example) and disadvantages (such as obesity and diabetes resulting from the combination of high-energy diets and sedentary living). However, an indication of how fragile the new system is, is the damage caused by

Cyclone Kina in Fiji in 1993. Fiji is one of the most economically developed countries in the Pacific, but Kina caused deaths, injuries, and massive economic losses. The production and distribution of food was severely affected. Following the cyclone, approximately 15 per cent of the national population (total 750 000 people) was dependent on food aid, for periods of up to three months (Olsthoorn *et al.* 1999).

Relative contributions of population size and economic activity to carbon dioxide emissions

The impact of humankind on the environment is a multiplicative function of three main variables: population size, level of material wealth (consumption), and types of technology. The potential multiplier from foreseeable population increase may now have become smaller than the potential multiplier due to changes in levels of economic activity – assuming no radical changes in technology. It seems that we are beginning to pass the peak rate of population increase, and the rate of addition of successive billions will slow until a stationary, or contracting, state is reached (Raleigh 1999). On the current 'median estimate', world population will increase by around another 3–4 billion over the coming century – that is, by a factor of about 1.6 relative to today's population of six billion. Meanwhile, if average global income (currently about US$5000/person/year) were to increase to the level of today's rich countries (currently about US$25 000/person/year) global economic product would multiply by a factor of five.

The ongoing climate change debate illustrates well the relative effects of population and consumption levels. During the twentieth century, the rate of carbon dioxide emissions from fossil fuel combustion increased 12-fold – the multiplicative result of a 3.5-fold increase in population and a 3.5-fold increase in per capita emission of carbon dioxide (Holdren 1991; Carbon Dioxide Information Analysis Centre 1997). For the coming century, it has been estimated that population growth will contribute around one-third of the increase in carbon dioxide emissions, whereas economic development will account for the remaining two-thirds (Bongaarts 1992). The economic development scenarios currently being used by the UN's IPCC to forecast global emissions of carbon dioxide entail 2- to 5-fold increases in global average income during the coming century (Carter and Hulme 1999).

To limit the carbon dioxide build-up to a doubling of its pre-industrial concentration (that is, from 275 ppm to 550 ppm) – a level which climatologists and ecologists think may be tolerable by most ecosystems – with a population of 10–11 billion by 2100, carbon dioxide emissions per person would need to be reduced to the levels of the 1920s (Carbon Dioxide Information Analysis Centre 1997; McMichael and Powles 1999; Wigley *et al.* 1996). That represents a reduction of approximately two-thirds from today's level. (The 1997 Kyoto Protocol was for an average five per cent cut relative to 1990 emission levels, and was restricted to developed countries.) If the more stringent, desirable, goal of 450 ppm were set, then humankind would need to achieve a 75 per cent reduction – taking emission levels back to those of 1900.

Difficulties in the scientific assessment of future health impacts

Scientists and policy makers do not, and will not, find it easy to assess and evaluate the risks posed to population health by this category of environmental change. To begin with, the empirical evidence implicating recent trends in regional and global climate in altered health outcomes is very thin. Indeed, more generally, our knowledge about how changes in climatic conditions affect a range of health outcomes is incomplete – and therefore leaves us a long way short of being able to predict the range, timing, and magnitude of various of the likely future health impacts of global environmental changes (McMichael 1997).

Further, the inevitable interaction between these processes, both as processes (for example the interplay between tropospheric warming and stratospheric cooling) and in their impacts on biophysical systems and on human populations, compounds the difficulty of predictive modelling. Considerable new scientific effort is now going into the development of integrated mathematical modelling, and into imbuing top-down models with the capacity for downscaled application to regions and countries, thereby taking account of local physical, ecological, and demographic particulars (McMichael *et al.* 2000*a*).

There is a particular challenge in dealing with uncertainties. Scenario-based risk assessment, especially in relation to complex processes and patterns of change, is an intrinsically uncertain exercise. Conventional quantitative risk assessment, based on observed risks in today's world and applied to existing population exposure profiles, can yield reasonable precision: statistical and situational uncertainties can often be greatly reduced. But forecasting future risks to health in a changed, and changeable, world entails many uncertainties. It is for this reason that the principle of *uncertainty-based* decision-making, in lieu of *risk-based* decision-making, is increasingly invoked in relation to this policy-making area.

The Precautionary Principle, as enunciated at the 1992 UN Conference on Environment and Development (the Rio 'Earth Summit'), thus becomes important. Where knowledge is uncertain and the situation complex, and where there is a finite – even if small – risk of serious, perhaps irreversible, damage to population health (or other socially valued outcome), then preventive action should be taken. Such preventive policies must be taken within a framework of 'uncertainty-based' (as opposed to a more empirically-grounded 'risk-based') assessment of possible outcomes.

Impediments to understanding and political action

As discussed above, meeting the needs of the current total world population, with prevailing technologies, results in the depletion of global stocks of resources and the overloading of environmental 'sinks' (Loh *et al.* 1998; McMichael *et al.* 2000*b*). This is an unprecedented crossroads for humankind to have reached, with great implications for the future levels and sustainability of human population health (McMichael and Powles 1999). Resolution will require more than just a few clever technical fixes (such as the rehabilitation of nuclear power generation and the worldwide diffusion of genetically modified higher-yielding crops). While such technological advances will relieve pressures temporarily, simple arithmetic shows that we will need a generalized radical 'greening' of our technologies – such as, for example, to reduce global carbon dioxide emissions by at least two-thirds (McMichael and Powles 1999).

To solve these large-scale 'common property problems' will require extraordinary levels of collective, equitable action. Social scientists regard that type of co-operation as intrinsically difficult for human societies to achieve (Caldwell 1990). Human communities generally find it difficult to achieve co-operation whenever substantive changes in social priorities, cultural values, and technological modes are required. This difficulty has been well illustrated by the complex forging – and the aftermath – of the Kyoto Protocol. This international protocol commits developed countries to making small cuts (five per cent on average) in their national emissions of carbon dioxide.

In responding to the threat of global environmental changes, supra-national collective action must overcome the self-interested rigidities of national sovereignty, strong vested corporate interests, cultural diversity, the grievances of the very poor against the minority of the very rich in an increasingly unequal world, and today's dominant philosophies of neo-liberalism, individual rights and the market place as rational arbiter of social choices. Caldwell, an historian, has observed of this particular contemporary challenge: 'The co-operative task would require behaviour that humans find most difficult: collective self-discipline in a common effort' (Caldwell 1990).

In this regard, it is important to note that the global environmental problem of stratospperic ozone depletion may well turn out to be 'the exception'. It appears that it can be substantially rectified by substitution of particular ozone-destroying gases used industrially and commercially. Even if that substitution is effectively achieved (there are still some technical and political problems), as mentioned above it has become evident more recently that warming in the lower atmosphere itself increases the autocatalytic destruction of stratospheric ozone. Nevertheless, compared to the other global environmental changes, replacing ozone-destroying gases is relatively straightforward, and does not require radical social, economic, or technological change. Further, the benefit of taking preventive action accrues within the immediate future, meaning that there is no problem of long-term deferral of time-discounted gains. The costs incurred can therefore be more readily justified within a conventional economic-political framework. This is one important difference from the question of greenhouse gas emission mitigation and its profile and schedule of costs and benefits.

The Kyoto Protocol: national reductions in greenhouse gas emissions

The Kyoto Protocol was agreed in November 1997 under the UN Framework Convention on Climate Change. It limits national emissions of greenhouse gases by the high-income (Annex I) countries. The protocol also laid the foundation for mitigation measures to reduce carbon dioxide emissions, including the provision for the international trading of carbon emission entitlements. The Kyoto Protocol will only become legally binding when at least 55 countries, including developed countries that account for at least 55 per cent of developed country emissions, have ratified. By late 2000, the protocol had been ratified by only a minority of countries. Several of the countries with highest per capita emissions, such as the USA, Canada, and Australia, have resisted early ratification, in contrast to the countries of Europe and Japan.

The protocol lists the prescribed reduction in carbon dioxide emissions that each individual country must achieve by the period 2008–2012 as a percentage of its 1990 levels: for example the USA (seven per cent), the European Union (eight per cent), the Russian Federation and Ukraine (zero per cent), Japan (six per cent). The achievement of these very modest goals (relative to what is required to actually stabilize atmospheric composition) is proving difficult. For example, during the 1990s the US carbon dioxide emissions have already increased, relative to 1990 emissions, by around one-seventh. Further, by the late 1990s only two, relatively small, non-industrialized countries had accepted any obligations.

The Kyoto Protocol, while of great political symbolic significance, falls far short of a prescription for curbing carbon dioxide emissions either worldwide or to a sufficient extent. In this it resembles the Montreal Protocol of 1987, which required substantive amendment in the 1990s to ensure that it actually achieved its ozone-protecting goal. As argued above, high-income countries will have to accept greater carbon dioxide emissions reduction, and low-income countries and countries in transition – 'whose legitimate growth and development interests must be recognized internationally – must also participate in emissions constraint, if not mitigation.

Because carbon dioxide emissions come from diverse sources such as industry, traffic, and households, there are many possible interventions. The Kyoto Protocol contains three 'flexible' instruments for international co-operative action:

+ tradable emissions permits (financial transactions in which each country has an agreed level of emission of greenhouse gases and a country exceeding its limit can 'buy' a quota of emissions from one that is emitting less)
+ the clean development mechanism (CDM)
+ joint implementation (JI) schemes

The case for tradable permits is based on the perceived advantages that it would offer relative to other politically feasible alternatives. It offers the possibility of reaching the environmental goals at a lower cost than if each country were limited to reducing emissions within its own borders. Making it easier to reach the goals may allow more countries to sign up to, and comply with, the Kyoto Protocol.

The latter two instruments allow joint emissions-reduction projects between high-income and low-income countries. The central principle is that high-income countries entering into joint emissions reductions programmes within low-income countries, would be credited with part of these reductions in lieu of domestic reductions. In practice, there is still much to do to determine which types of projects would qualify and what should be the respective roles and credits of the participating states. Approved joint schemes might include investments in reforestation, the upgrading of energy generation facilities, installation of emissions-control technologies in states such as China and India, and protecting the rain forest in Brazil. Such initiatives would lead, in effect, to the international co-financing of international standards in the field of the environment.

Via these flexible mechanisms, there is hope that countries would develop a better understanding of the advantages of global co-operation and of the co-financing of development. More ambitiously, it may open the door to eventually extending the mechanisms to allow for measures such as investing in education, investing in means that have a positive effect of reducing birth rates, introducing information and communications technologies, and so on. Eventually, these Kyoto-type mechanisms, especially the CDM, might lead to an international process in which the rights for limited pollution options are distributed around the globe, beginning with a 'grandfather-type' distribution, and evolving to equal distribution per person.

Important questions include the following.

(1) Are tradable permits a useful tool for achieving a global reduction of greenhouse gas emissions? Which are the key steps for implementing tradable permits (benchmarks)?

(2) What will be the ecological effect of transferring resources to the South? What will be the costs per carbon dioxide reduction unit of these transfer measures, compared to costs of achieving further restrictive standards in high-income countries?

(3) Can the transaction costs involved in determining and transferring the rights among countries and between the public and private sectors be satisfactorily modelled?

Information and communication technologies will play a key role in achieving sustainable development that favours efficient use of materials and energy. However, there is always the risk that those technologies will result in unintended 'rebound effects' due to higher levels of consumption in response to the efficiency-related lower unit prices. Therefore, an appropriate worldwide policy framework, supported by newly adopted values and attitudes, must also be achieved to avert rebound effects.

The contribution of health professionals

In considering what health professionals can do, it may be helpful to reflect on responses to earlier environmental crises. Climate change and ozone depletion result from 'overload' at a global scale. In the nineteenth century it was local systems for disposal of human and industrial waste that were overwhelmed by the rapid concentration of large populations in cities and the expansion of manufacturing operations. Health professionals contributed in a number of ways to understanding and controlling the adverse effects of industrialization and urban growth. In the UK, medical officers of health collected data on numbers and causes of death that were the basis of influential reports such as Chadwick's *Report on the sanitary conditions of the labouring classes*. Doctors (and nurses – Florence Nightingale's contribution to public health should not be overlooked) were responsible in large part for translating the vision of the sanitary reformers into effective, practical programmes (Porter 1999). John Simon and other 'doctors-turned-statesman' took their arguments directly to senior politicians. Others established advocacy groups, such as the Metropolitan Health of Towns Association created by Southwood Smith in 1844, that attempted to influence public opinion more widely.

The next phase of environmental health was concerned with control of specific physical and chemical hazards, not necessarily confined to national or even regional boundaries. Health professionals took prominent roles here also, individually and collectively, in response to widespread pollutants such as lead, tobacco, and asbestos. These roles included research, public education, and lobbying.

The International Physicians for Prevention of Nuclear War (IPPNW) is perhaps the first environmental health example of concerted action at an international level. This group was formed in 1981, and aimed to capitalize on the esteem with which doctors are generally regarded, the knowledge that they hold of the medical consequences of radiation and war, the international networks of the profession, and the personal connections with persons of influence. (The co-chair of IPPNW was for some years personal physician to the President of the Soviet Union.) IPPNW was active in education, lobbying, and direct approaches to the leaders of major powers. The numbers of doctors involved grew rapidly, the group was rewarded with the Nobel Prize for peace in 1985, and according to the testimony of one senior figure (Mikhail Gorbachev), the efforts of IPPNW did indeed make a difference to policies on nuclear weapons (Lown 1988).

With these examples in mind, we suggest that health professionals can contribute to the control of global environmental problems in three ways. First, they have an essential role to play as technicians, as people who understand the ways in which environmental influences can affect human health and are experienced in assessing evidence. In this capacity health professionals act as advisors to international and national agencies, governments, private industry, and non-governmental organizations. Second, as opinion-leaders, health professionals have a responsibility to connect their specialist knowledge with common understanding. Finally, where health is seriously at risk, health professionals must act also as advocates, which means engaging in social action. This may seem remote from the primary activity of most health workers, but as we have already indicated, there is a long history of doctors and other health professionals involving themselves in social and political struggles that concern health. In this instance, the challenge of environmental threats is global in scale, and so the social and political struggles to overcome these threats will also be global, and international co-operation will be essential.

Conclusion

We have emphasized the point that climate change and stratospheric ozone depletion are two examples of a new kind of environmental threat. This threat is the consequence of overload and breakdown of global homeostatic mechanisms. Climate change and ozone depletion illustrate a simple and inescapable truth: the planet is a closed system. Problems like these that are inherently global in nature require a response that is also worldwide. This means that international co-operation will be even more important that in the past, when diseases may have been distributed globally, but the causes were essentially local.

John Houghton, former chair of the IPCC, has proposed that international agreements to deal with global environmental issues such as climate change should be based on three principles (Houghton 1999). These include the Precautionary Principle, which states that if a threat is potentially serious, then scientific uncertainty does not justify inaction. The second is the Polluter Pays Principle, implying that the full environmental cost of pollution should be borne by those responsible. The third principle, and possibly the most contentious, is that of equity. Considerations of equity or fairness apply between countries and over time. The balance of benefits and costs of climate change, for example, is likely to differ between affluent communities in the north and marginal populations in the south, and between current generations (who may benefit from early stages of warming) and future generations (for whom costs will outweigh benefits, if forecast warming trends continue).

It will not be straightforward to apply these principles in practice, given the difficulties of assessing 'serious' threats, allocating costs accurately, and agreeing on definitions of fairness. However, there is no reason to believe that the challenge is an impossible one. Although imperfect, the Montreal Protocol provided an example of how international agreements can proceed in the face of uncertainty. In the case of climate change, specific suggestions have been made on how considerations of equity and 'polluter pays' can be translated into policy. The UK-based Global Commons Institute, for example, has developed a 'contraction and convergence' framework for allocating future tradable emissions, on the basis that countries with the highest emissions take the sharpest reductions in quota, with the ultimate goal (by 2100) being equality of per capita shares worldwide in greenhouse gas emissions.

These issues loom large to all of us – health professionals and everyone else. We are all citizens in an emerging global constituency that now faces unprecedented global-level common-property problems. Since those environmental changes portend new risks to population health, there is an important role for health professionals to play, everywhere, in helping to elucidate, communicate, and respond to these issues.

References

Bongaarts, J. (1992) Population growth and global warming. *Population and Development Review,* **18,** 299–319.

Briguglio, L. (1993) Small island states and their economic vulnerabilities. *World Development,* February, 1615–32.

Caldwell, L. (1990) *Between two worlds.* Cambridge University Press, Cambridge.

Cameron, J. (1997) Public policy for a better nourished healthier South Pacific population consistent with sustainable environments and ecologies. In *Environment and development in the Pacific Islands,* ed. B. Burt and C. Clerk, pp. 216–38. National Centre for Development Studies, Australian National University, Canberra.

Campbell, J. R. (1999) Pacific island vulnerabilities towards the end of the twentieth century. In *natural disaster management. A presentation to commemorate the international decade for natural disaster reduction 1999–2000,* ed. J. Ingelton, pp. 90–3. Tudor Rose, London.

Carbon Dioxide Information Analysis Centre (1997) *Historical carbon dioxide emissions.* Oak Ridge National Laboratory, Oak Ridge, TN.

Carter, T. and Hulme, M. (1999) Interim characterizations of regional climate and related changes up to 2100 associated with the SRES emissions scenarios, draft report. Intergovernmental Panel on Climate Change, Geneva.

Department of Health (2000) *Potential health impacts of climate change in the UK.* Department of Health, London.

Downing, T. E. and Bakker, K. (1999) Drought vulnerability: concepts and theory. In *Drought*, ed. D. A. Wilhite. Routledge, New York.

Drager, N. (1999) Making trade work for public health. *British Medical Journal*, **319**, 1214.

Dyson, T. (1999) Prospects for feeding the world. *British Medical Journal*, **319**, 988–91.

Focks, D., Daniels, D. G., Haile, D. G. *et al.* (1995) A simulation model of epidemiology of urban dengue: literature analysis, model development, preliminary validation and samples of simulation results. *American Journal of Tropical Medicine and Hygiene*, **53**, 489–506.

Folke, C., Larsson, J. and Sweitzer, J. (1996) Renewable resource appropriation. In *Getting down to earth*, ed. R. Costanza and O. Segura. Island Press, Washington DC.

FAO (1995) *State of the world's fisheries.* Food and Agricultural Organization, Rome.

FAO (1999) *Food insecurity.* Food and Agricultural Organization, Rome.

Greenland, D. J., Gregory, P. J., and Nye, P. H. (1998) Land resources and constraints to crop production. In: *Feeding a world population of more than eight billion people*, ed. J. C. Waterlow, D. G. Armstrong, L. Fowden, R. Riley, pp. 39–55. Oxford University Press, Oxford.

Holdren, J. P. (1991) Population and the energy problem. *Population and Environment*, **12**, 231–55.

Houghton, J. (1999) As things hot up. *The Economist:The World in 2000*, December, 146.

Houghton, J. T., Meira Filho, L. G., Callander, B. A. *et al.* (1995) Climate change, 1995 – the science of climate change: contribution of working group I to the second assessment report of the Intergovernmental Panel on Climate Change. Cambridge University Press, Cambridge.

IPCC (in press) Chapter 14 (Health). In *Special report on technology transfer.*

Kaly, U., Briguglio, L., McLeod, H. *et al.* (1999) Enviromental vulnerability index (EVI) to summarise national environmental vulnerability profiles. SOPAC Technical Report 275. South Pacific Applied Geoscience Commission (SOPAC), Suva, Fiji.

Levins, R. (1995) Preparing for uncertainty. *Ecosystem Health*, **1**, 47–57.

Loh, J., Randers, J., MacGillivray, A. *et al.* (1998) Living planet report. WWF International, Gland, Switzerland.

Lown, B. (1988) Looking back, seeing ahead. *Lancet*, **ii**, 203–4.

Martens, W. J. M. (1998) *Health and climate change: modelling the impacts of global warming and ozone depletion.* Earthscan, London.

Martens, W. J. M., Kovats, R. S., Nijhof, S. *et al.* (1999) Climate change and future populations at risk of malaria. *Global Environmental Change*, **9** (suppl.), S89–107.

McMichael, A. J. (1993) *Planetary overload. global environmental change and the health of the human species.* Cambridge University Press, Cambridge.

McMichael, A. J. (1997) Integrated assessment of potential health impact of global environmental change: prospects and limitations. *Environmental Modelling and Assessment*, **2**, 129–37.

McMichael, A. J. and Haines, A. (1997) Climate change and potential impacts on human health. *British Medical Journal*, **315**, 805–9.

McMichael, A. J. and Powles, J. W. P. (1999) Human numbers, environment, sustainability and health. *British Medical Journal*, **319**, 977–80.

McMichael, A. J., Haines, A., Slooff, R. *et al.* (1996) Climate change and human health (WHO/EHG/96.7). WHO, Geneva.

McMichael, A. J., Martens, W. J. M., Lele, S. *et al.* (2000*a*) Methods of assessing the health impact of climate change. In *Disease and exposure mapping*, ed. P. Elliott, J. C. Wakefield, N.G. Best, *et al.*, pp. 444–461. Oxford University Press, Oxford.

McMichael, A. J., Smith, K. R. and Corvalan, C. (2000*b*) The sustainable transition: a new challenge. *Bulletin of the World Health Organisation*, **78**, 1067.

Meyer, W. B. (1996) *Human impact on the Earth.* Cambridge University Press, Cambridge.

Olsthoorn, A. A., Maunder, W. J., and Tol, R. S. J. (1999) Tropical cyclones in the southwest Pacific: impacts on Pacific island countries with particular reference to Fiji. In *Climate Change and Risk*, ed. T. E. Downing, A. J. Olsthoorn and R. S. J. Tol, pp. 221–44. Routledge, London.

Parry, M. L. and Rosenzweig, C. (1993) Food supply and risk of hunger. *Lancet,* **342**, 1345–7.

Pollock, N. J. (1992) *These roots remain. Food habits in islands of the central and eastern Pacific since western Contact.* University of Hawaii Press, Honolulu.

Porter, D. (1999) *Health, civilization and the state. A history of public health from ancient to modern times.* Routledge, London.

Raleigh, V. S. (1999) World population and health in transition. *British Medical Journal*, **319**, 981–4.

Schep, J. (1997) International trade for local development: the case for western Solomon Islands fair trade. In *Environment and development in the Pacific Islands*, ed. B. Burt and C. Clerk, pp. 78–90. National Centre for Development Studies, Australian National University, Canberra.

Sen, A. (1981) *Poverty and famines: an essay on entitlement and deprivation.* Clarendon Press, Oxford.

Shindell, D. T., Rind, D., and Lonergan, P. (1998) Increased polar stratospheric ozone losses and delayed eventual recovery owing to increasing greenhouse gas concentrations. *Nature*, **392**, 589–92.

Slaper, H., Velders, G. J. M., Daniel, J. S. *et al.* (1996) Estimates of ozone depletion and skin cancer incidence to examine the Vienna Convention achievements. *Nature*, **384**, 256–8.

UNEP (1998) Environmental effects of ozone depletion. 1998 assessment. Elsevier, Lausanne.

Vitousek, P. M., Mooney, H. A., Lubchenco, J. *et al.* (1997) Human domination of Earth's ecosystems. *Science*, **277**, 494–9.

Wackernagel, M. and Rees, W. (1995) *Our ecological footprint. reducing human impact on the earth.* New Society Publishers, Gabriola Island, BC Canada.

Wang, X. and Smith, K. R. (2000) Secondary benefits of greenhouse gas control: health impact in China. *Environmental Science Technology*, **33**, 3056–61.

Watson, R. T., Dixon, J. A., Hamburg, S. P. *et al* (1998) Protecting our planet. Securing our future. Linkages among global environmental issues and human needs. UNEP/USNASA/World Bank.

WHO (1999) World health report. WHO, Geneva.

Wigley, T. M. L., Richels, R., and Edmonds, J. A. (1996) Economic and environmental choices in the stabilization of atmospheric CO2 concentrations. *Nature*, **379**(18), 240–3.

Woodward, A., Hales, S., and Weinstein, P. (1998) Climate change and human health in the Asia Pacific: who will be most vulnerable? *Climate Research*, **11**, 31–8.

Working Group on Public Health and Fossil-Fuel Combustion (1997) Short-term improvements in public health and global climate policies on fossil fuel combustion: an interim report. *Lancet*, **350**, 1341–9.

World Bank (1997) World development report, the state in a changing world. IBRD, Washington DC.

World Commission on Environment and Development (1987) *Our common future*. Oxford University Press, Oxford.

Chapter 6

Trade, public health, and food

Tim Lang

Introduction

Since 1950, gross world production has increased five-fold, but world trade has increased fourteen-fold. For proponents of trade, this is an astonishing success story. Economists and politicians often cite such statistics as evidence that trade is now the motor force not just of the global economy but of human progress itself. According to this reading of the contemporary political economy, trade is an unalloyed good with direct benefits for health.

The case for a positive interpretation may be summarized thus: more trade leads to more wealth, which in turn improves health. While it is undoubtedly true that wealthier people live longer and tend to have lives less plagued by ill health, the relationship between trade and health can be deceptive. The uni-linear relationship proposed by the positive interpretation of trade and health in fact covers a multitude of dynamics. That is why this chapter takes a more sober look at the role of trade and its implications for public health. It argues in particular that the relationship between trade and health is both complex and problematic. Changing patterns of disease, methods of production, and control mean that key issues are raised for Public Health, to such an extent that our notion of what public health practice is must change.

This chapter takes food as its core illustrations, so the arguments offered are subject to a caveat. It is possible that some of the issues discussed here are peculiar to the food sector. However, food is so important that even if the arguments explored here are specific to food, then they deserve to be taken seriously. After all, food is a basic human need without which good health is impossible and also a basic right under the United Nations (UN) Declaration of Human Rights, agreed by governments since 1948. Issues covered in this chapter, such as governance and the use of energy, have direct relevance beyond food policy. The perspective taken here is in line with the World Health Organization (WHO) analysis that health is socially determined (Marmot and Wilkinson 1998; Wilkinson 1996). This is not to deny the immense importance of genes; far from it, but pending any dramatic – and ethically momentous – shift into mass genetic engineering, our attention in public health will mainly be on the social characteristics of human life and on public policy interventions to tackle social conditions. These are the key variables that public health professions and interventions can alter. The focus in this chapter is therefore on these features rather than on the fascinating implications of the new discoveries about the interplay of genes and nutrients (Barker 1992).

Raising public health questions about food and trade

In 1994, the signing of a new General Agreement on Tariffs and Trade (GATT) brought public health into the trade area almost without people in public health realizing it, even though trade specialists were already somewhat nervous about the potential of health considerations to destabilize neo-liberal trade theory (Lang 1992). Within a few years, the five areas of agriculture, biodiversity, health standards, technical barriers to trade, and trade in services had raised public health concerns and the public health world was beginning to be involved in a self-education process. Sparked by active educational and lobbying work by non-governmental organizations (NGOs), many health researchers and bodies began to take an active interest in trade. A critical literature began to swell (Kim *et al.* 2000; Koivusalo 1999; Labonte 1998; Lang 1999a; Taylor and Thomas 1999), but once again, NGOs took the lead. At Seattle in December 1999, the world's civil society met in a vast, well organized series of meetings, lobbying, and street action, all designed to pressurize the talks to revise the GATT. Now under the aegis of the newly formed World Trade Organization (WTO), the trade talks came to a halt for a host of reasons, which vary according to perspective. They range from concerns about trade priorities, EU–USA tensions, north–south splits over democracy, and Machiavellian internal US politics to general criticisms that the WTO and GATT are too favourable to big business, anti-environment, weak on animal protection and undemocratic.

Seattle was an astonishing event, transforming the whole trade debate from a political backwater for policy specialists into world news. In certain areas, such as the Agreement on Agriculture, trade negotiations continued having their own timetable, but in the main, Seattle bought some breathing space and opportunities for civic society to consider its options. Public health too has its obligations to participate openly in this world debate. How can this be translated for food policy? A series of questions can be formulated.

Firstly, although the food sector is currently subject to the most astonishing changes – new products, technologies, processes, and distribution channels – the public health message about food is in fact pretty clear (Cannon 1992). Both global and national reports on food and health stress the fact that global disease patterns are now dominated by diet-related degenerative diseases such as heart disease, cancers, and diabetes (Comission on the Nutrition Challenges of the 21st Century 2000). More is always being learned about the aetiology of these diseases, but the broad parameters seem pretty clear. The constituents of a diet that is protective for health is broadly known (WHO 1990). It has to be sufficient and rich in key nutrients. It is likely to be high in fruit and vegetables, low in total fats, high in cereals. Yet when we look at what people eat around the world the trends are away from such a diet. The questions we have to ask of trade are: is trade involved in this process? And is it a benign or malignant force?

Secondly, alongside the degenerative diseases, there also exist more 'traditional' but man-made problems of underconsumption. The simple historical truth is that there is enough food to feed the world, if one applies a notion of nutritional adequacy (Alexandros 1995). The problem, however, is that this total supply sufficiency is not equitably shared. As a result, the world food situation is now dominated by simultaneous malnourishment and overconsumption. A UN report in 2000 could conclude of both developing and undeveloped countries having a 'fundamental link between maternal and early child undernutrition and an increased susceptibility in adult life to non-communicable diseases such as diabetes, heart disease and hypertension'. . . and that these are 'already major public health challenges for developing countries' (Commission on the Nutrition Challenges of the 21st Century 2000). The question to ask now is whether in this context, trade is feeding the needy or the greedy or both.

Thirdly, turning to public policy on food, there is now a consensus that policy ought to be based on what we might call the four pillars of public health: food safety, nutrition, social justice, and environmental health (it can be argued that in public policy, the last two are merged into one under the heading 'sustainable development' but for our purposes here, it is useful to disaggregate people from the planet). Yet almost everywhere in the world, food safety dominates political and policy attention. The key politicians, those concerned with economics, see food safety as a 'spoiler' factor, something that requires more expenditure but on which consumers are increasingly demanding. It is not hard to see why food safety now looms large for trade. It poses serious problems, undermining public confidence and introducing volatility when what is sought is stability. The question here is: are trade policies giving the right messages towards health or are they either overnarrow or, worse, dismissive? For instance, by encouraging people to eat more fish (for their essential fats), are nutritionists unwittingly contributing to environmental damage from overfishing?

Fourthly, there is an issue of trade and culture. It is now widely accepted that health is socially determined to a significant degree. Food is no exception to this general rule. Any observer of contemporary food culture is struck by the coincidence of two features. An astonishing legacy of culinary and dietary diversity is being affected by a rapid process of globalization. Globo-food is quietly replacing more local and traditional foods. Does this matter? Are the benefits of choice giving enough health gain to compensate for historical or cultural perceived loss? Are people in control of the process of change or are they being controlled by it?

Fifthly, institutions of governance are now subject to extraordinary pressures. Fierce critics and proponents of globalization both argue that national governments need to change. A global economy has replaced national economies, thereby rendering local governance obsolete. For public health, the issue is not just whether this analysis is true but whether it matters. Are the institutions which mediate between consumer and food supply appropriate to rise to the health challenge? Is the WTO, for instance, usurping the UN? What, in short, is the challenge of globalization to public health governance?

These are all immensely complex questions to which sometimes no exact or definitive answers can be given but the questions have to be posed and explored. Public policy is made with or without good answers. Politics does not wait for researchers! One among many challenges for public health professionals is to take a more active role in the policy process at the same time as trying to grapple with the intellectual implications of these issues.

With these large-scale questions in mind, what is the relationship between trade and health that emerges from food?

This chapter argues that the relationship between food, trade, and health is complex, and always has been. It argues that the current dynamics and drivers of the food economy marginalize health. It notes, in particular, that globally there is a transition from a more local/national and simple diet to a more complex and globally traded one and that this transition carries costs, rarely acknowledged by proponents of global food trade. These costs arise at a number of levels including human health, environmental health, geographical, economic, and social. The analysis concludes that to make public health anything other than marginal in trade policy, and to deliver food security in a world which is rapidly urbanizing and fragmenting, there will have to be a considerable rethink about food governance as well as the direction of food policy.

The complex relationship between food, trade, and health

Public policy has an immense challenge in grappling with the relationship between food, trade, and health. It is complex and always has been, but changes to the food economy, which are explored below, have made that relationship even more complex.

Food is essential for health. Its absence leads not just to food insecurity but heralds ill health and, at its most extreme, death. The role of trade in mediating this double-edged relationship is central. As a primary commodity, food is and always has been central to trade and exchange (Smith 1995). Through this transfer, humanity's capacity to feed itself and make or break its health has been transformed.

For centuries, crop specialization, whether due to favourable terrain, climate, or skill, has meant that surpluses have been available for trade. As biodiversity has spread, so have the possibilities of improved nutrition and health. One just has to consider the impact of the dissemination of the potato from Peru or wheat from the middle east throughout the world to realize that humans have gained immense advantages from culinary diversity. But health is not the only aspect of human life affected by food trade.

Food, while carrying this promise of better health, also offers opportunities for economic and social control. World food statistics show that food is in surplus (Food and Agriculture Organization (FAO) 1999) but that good access is prevented by poor distribution, unequal income, and politics. Famines teach us that entitlement is not the same thing as a full belly (Sen and Dreze 1981). Trade is an opportunity to make money and a means for social status. Tastes and cultural predilections for foods are made, not given. It was ever thus. In ancient Greece, and particularly classical Athens, social relations could be tracked not just by what was eaten but by whom (Dalby 1996). The tomato may have a treasured place within Italian cuisine today but in fact it is an arriviste from across the Atlantic only five centuries ago, a product of the so-called Columbian exchange when Europe annexed the Americas. One era's delicacies can become its successor's normal food.

To a cook, in theory, trade can be a boon, liberating the stove from seasonality, but it is surprising how often cookery pundits celebrate the local and the fresh. Fresh foods from the other hemisphere in one's mid winter are the culinary equivalent of a mid-winter trip to the sun, a marvellous tonic but generally available only to the affluent! Although transfers between the hemispheres catch the eye as we browse in our local retail stores, historically transfers have tended to be broadly along the same latitudes, for climatic reasons. The Arabs, for instance, spread oranges westwards to the Mediterranean (Bianchini *et al.* 1988); today they are common throughout Europe and the world. But the oldest foods to be traded tended to be dry or easily stored. Salt, above all, has been a prized traded commodity (Adshead 1992), a preservative extraordinaire, an excess of which is now associated with hypertension. Coffee, cocoa, sugar, tea, spices, potatoes, and tomatoes, have all travelled far from their botanical origins, their so-called Vavilov centres (named after Vavilov, the Russian scientist who mapped geographical origins of seeds), usually as a result of colonial trading relations. In the last half millennium, these plants became global commodities (Rowling 1987; Winson 1993).

These cases enable us to note that the impact of the food trade on health is not just a direct one through the *physical* transfer of commodities but also one of *ideas* and *culture* – a cuisine, a way of growing a product, an expectation of what food is. In Britain, for example, pizza (Italian) and curries (Indian) are now routine items on menus, and modern children think of them as British just as their grandparents conceived them as foreign or exotic.

Health's place among the food economy's current drivers and dynamics

The exploration of food and trade is a fascinating subject and rightly a rich site for historical investigation (Adshead 1992; Hobhouse 1985; Mintz 1985), but what of its health implications? Diet is a key factor in many sources of ill health, ranging from degenerative diseases such as coronary heart disease and some cancers to communicable diseases through food contamination. Food's role in health is again double-edged: it can be both a main cause of ill health and a key factor in prevention. It is this role of trade in enabling food to be either a positive or a negative health factor that has brought trade to the forefront of modern debates about health in that the dominant policy approach to trade is to encourage it in the name of liberalization and globalization.

At the end of the twentieth century, there was considerable debate about globalization (Castells 1996; Scholte 2000). The impression was given that this was something completely new. Food gives the lie to that view. The shifting of foods around the world has been going on for millennia. What is new today, however, is the pace, the scale and who controls that change (see also Chapter 2). It is more accurate therefore to talk of different *phases* or *eras* of globalization and to note that the modern era has ushered in new methods for food trade and a new and systematic manner for exerting control over foods (Lang 1999b).

Globalization and regionalization

Much food eaten around the world is still nationally or regionally produced but there is a tendency for food exports to rise, accelerated by high degrees of concentration in national home markets, a process which encourages food economies to shift from local or national to regional supply chains. Rather than focus just on globalization, more attention ought also to be paid by public health to *regionalization.* Heffernan and colleagues, for instance, have shown how US agribusiness has consolidated into three core groupings or constellations of companies (Heffernan 1999). We shall see below how large food companies, even though hugely powerful by historical terms, are still far from controlling entire world markets. Nestlé, for instance, the world's largest food company still only sells 1.8 per cent of world food.

The emergence of huge intranational regional trade blocs is one of the key economic characteristics of the post-World War 2 period. The emergence of the EU, Asia Pacific Economic Co-operation (APEC), Mercosur, the Association of South East Asian Nations (ASEAN) and even the residual groupings left over from the former Soviet Union, all point in the same historical direction – the *transnationalization* of food trade.

The nutrition and health transition

What makes the issue of trade so important for health policy – and all public policy – is a phenomenon known as the nutrition transition. Centuries-old diets are being altered comparatively speedily in a process Popkin and co-workers have termed the nutrition transition (Drewnoski and Popkin 1997; Popkin 1994). This thesis, which global data support, argues simply that diet-related ill health previously associated with the west and with affluence is now manifest in developing countries. While Popkin argues that the transition might bring greater variety to people who have narrow diets, the problems cannot and should not be traded off against the gains. Public health requires whole populations to improve.

Data support the thesis. The WHO World Health Report, for instance, shows that certain food-related cancers are increasing worldwide (WHO 1999). Different types of cancers feature in the south than in the north. In the south there are more cancers of the oesophagus, liver, and cervix. In the north, there is a predominance of cancers of the lung, colon, pancreas, and breast. The good news is that coronary heart disease (CHD) is declining in the north after years of growth. The bad news is that CHD is now emerging in the south, particularly among the more affluent classes who are adopting a western lifestyle and dietary attributes. They are consuming more meat and dairy fats, salt, and sugary foods and drinks, and fewer cereals and legumes, and taking less exercise.

In the middle east, the WHO has reported that changing diets and lifestyles with urbanization are now resulting in changing patterns of mortality and morbidity (Verster 1996). In Saudi Arabia, for instance, meat consumption doubled and fat consumption tripled between the mid–1970s and early 1990s. Jordan has seen a sharp rise in deaths from cardiovascular disease. But these problems sit alongside protein–energy malnutrition, especially among children. A huge study of diet and health within China found evidence of the nutrition transition in that as the population in the sample urbanized, its health profile began to follow a more western pattern of diet-related disease (Chen *et al.* 1990). Its diet altered, with the replacement of legumes such as soya bean by animal protein in the form of meat. As a result, degenerative diseases became more prevalent.

The Global Burden of Disease Study (Murray and Lopez 1997) provides an insight into the causes of death relevant to diet. This study was a detailed review of all causes of mortality for eight regions of the world. It identified the 30 leading causes of global mortality in 1990. Ischaemic heart disease was the leading cause of death worldwide, accounting for 6.26 million deaths, 2.7 million were in established market economies and former socialist economies of Europe, 3.6 million were in developing countries (out of 50.5 million deaths from all causes in 1990). Stroke was the next most common cause of death (4.38 million, almost 3 million in developing countries), closely followed by acute respiratory infections (4.3 million, 3.9 million in developing countries). Other leading cause of death include diarrhoeal disease (almost totally in developing countries), chronic obstructive pulmonary disease, tuberculosis, measles, low birthweight, road-traffic accidents, and lung cancer. With the exception of diarrhoea and low birthweight, none of these has a diet-related aetiology.

All cancers caused about 6 million deaths in 1990. About 2.4 million cancer deaths occurred in established market economies and former socialist economies of Europe. By 1990, therefore, there were already 50 per cent more cancer deaths in less developed countries than in developed countries.

One review of this problem concluded that exhortation to consume more soy when they were voting with their purses to eat more meat would be ineffective 'in the context of an increasingly free and global market' (Geissler 1999) The battle to prevent western diseases appears already to have been lost. It can be argued that health care systems, individuals, societies, and insurance companies are now paying the price for changes of which corporations are the prime financial beneficiaries.

The cultural transition

The nutrition transition is also a cultural transition. Rice eaters are becoming wheat eaters. People who previously ate meat rarely now associate meat with affluence and aspire to meat daily. In this process, food shifts from being a need to being a lifestyle product. Cooking occurs less in the home and more in factories or institutions (hotels, restaurants, cafés, canteens). This is why western burger chains are such cultural icons not just for globalizers but for health critics. In a comparatively short period, the world is experiencing a rapid transformation in basic diet. As a result, health-policy makers should recognize that when corporations mould taste, there is a health cost that they do not pay for (Barnet and Cavanagh 1994; Lang 1997; Mintz 1996). This is a tension reminiscent of the fight over tobacco and health.

Cultural flows can, of course, be two-way. Few affluent western societies have not been heavily influenced by immigrant foods: north African couscous in France, curries in Britain, Mexican food in the USA, pizzas and Chinese food everywhere. The more powerful flow in products is generally north to south, even while ideas may flow in the other direction. As processed food styles are exported from north to south, consumers in the developing world are encouraged to think of food and drink as coming not from farmers or the earth but from processed food corporations (Norberg-Hodge 1991). After a comparatively short exposure to western brands, the brand name of

Coca-Cola was recognized by 65 per cent of Chinese, Pepsi by 42 per cent, and Nestlé by 40 per cent (Gallup 1995).

Meat

A key feature of the new globalizing food culture is an acceleration of meat eating. One estimate is that meat consumption will grow 43 per cent worldwide by 2020, with an accompanying 40 per cent rise in demand for cereals to feed the animals (Commission on the Nutrition Challenges of the 21st Century 2000). Yet since 1950, the area per person available for grain harvest has declined from 0.23 hectares to 0.12 hectares by 1998 (Brown *et al.* 1999).

In China, according to the International Food Policy Research Institute (IFPRI), per capita demand for beef, poultry, and pig meat is set to double in the period 1993–2020. In many cultures, meat is associated with wealth (and festivals), yet meat is notoriously inefficient as a converter of energy. Crudely, it takes 7 kg of feed to produce 1 kg of feedlot-produced meat, 2 kg to produce 1 kg of poultry meat and 4 kg to produce 1 kg of pig meat (Rosegrant *et al.* 1999). According to FAO data, meat consumption is growing in developing countries at the rate of 4.7 per cent per year and in developed economies at the rate of 1.9 per cent per year. IFPRI, however, has calculated that a dramatic fall in meat consumption, by 50 per cent, would only deliver approximately 1 or 2 per cent decline in child malnourishment (Rosegrant *et al.* 1999). A curtailment of feeding animals in rich countries would not automatically be translated into improved diets for the poor in developing countries. It warns against over-simple solutions such as mass vegetarianism, although there is good evidence that such a diet can be entirely satisfactory for health (see the summary in Sanders 1999).

This complexity of trends suggests that perhaps the environmental and social cost of meat eating will have to be more central in public policy. Whatever the demand, the supply might not be freely available. Nutritionally, the warning signs are already well rehearsed. Western diets, high in animal and other fats and low in complex carbohydrates, have been shown to play a role in the so-called 'western' degenerative diseases (coronary heart disease, some cancers). With increased life expectancy the 'western' degenerative diseases are emerging in more significant numbers in cultures which lack the medical facilities to treat them (Commission on the Nutrition Challenges of the 21st Century 2000; Worldwatch Institute 2000).

Behind what appears to be local meat – or indeed any food – may lie a global operation. The product label may say 'produce of Brazil /USA /Japan', but there can be a global assembly process beneath the surface. An animal reared in Europe may have been fed on foods from around the world (Paxton 1994). Certain features of this process are critical for any understanding of globalization's public health implications. Only the rich can afford the exotic, but then when the exotic becomes mass market, margins fall and total revenues explode. This dynamic was central to the late twentieth century food globalization process. There is both a 'pull' – consumers aspiring to better their food lot – and a 'push' – companies seeking new markets.

Meat, for instance, is associated with wealth, so if cheaper meat is available, its connotations of affluence are available to more people. Another illustration of this cultural process has occurred with white bread. Prior to the invention of fast roller mills in the 19th century, white flour was the preserve of the rich. New fast mills allowed a niche market to become a mass market, making available the bran for animal food. Yet in health terms, of course, the whole wheat bread is better.

With meat sales suffering tighter margins, declining sales, and health criticism in affluent markets, meat producers in the USA, Europe and elsewhere have been desperate to expand meat markets overseas. In testimony to the US Congress in 1999, before the débacle at Seattle of the trade talks, the National Cattlemen's Beef Association gave a clear insight to how important exports were to the US meat sector (Lambert 1999):

> Exports of beef have helped to take up the slack of declining demand for beef at home. We as an industry have worked hard to promote beef exports which now account for over 12 per cent of the value of [US] wholesale beef sales. [. . .] The Seattle round of world trade talks will be the defining moment for world agricultural trade. The US beef industry has worked hard to expand sales of our product in the younger, fast growing, overseas market.

Moulding tastes

Besides its scale, speed, and global reach, a key characteristic of the new era of food globalization is the application of marketing techniques to the moulding of taste. This requires a merger of production and consumption using 'just-in-time' logistics. Examples are the manner in which burger culture has been introduced into Asia in the 1990s (Ritzer 1997, 1999), and the integration of production of fresh vegetables and fruit in developing countries where land and labour is cheap, with their selling in affluent markets of the west (Thruss 1995). Such 'efficiencies' of course are entirely dependent upon cheap fossil fuels for transportation. Without this, the joys of being able to drink French bottled water in the USA or to consume Brazilian orange juice in the middle of Australian citrus-growing areas, or to eat 'Greek' feta cheese in Greece which in fact was made in Denmark would be unthinkable.

The environmental transition

Human health is not the only factor in transition; so is environmental health. As we saw above, meat is a good illustration of how apparently 'efficient' food production systems may be environmentally wasteful. Intensive agriculture can use more energy in the form of non-renewable resources notably oil and also man-made fertilizers than is harvested in a form available for human food.

One study of the beef market, for instance, has suggested the emergence of the 'world steer', an animal reared in Latin America, using US feedlot technology, fed on European antibiotics, and marketed in Japan (Sanderson 1986). The hidden energy use – with costs externalized onto the environment – are only just beginning to emerge. Food needs to be judged not just by quality and price but by its food miles/kilometres, i.e. the distance it has travelled (Paxton 1994).

In the UK, 685 000 gigajoules of energy (equivalent to 14 million litres of fuel) were consumed in transporting the 417 207 tonnes of dessert apples imported into the UK in just one year, 1993 (Garnett 1999). Dessert apples can perfectly well be grown in the UK, and used to be until fruit farmers were 'encouraged' out of business by the European Union (EU) Common Agriculture Policy. According to the UK Department of Transport, despite approximately the same tonnage of food being consumed annually within the UK, over the last two decades the amount of food being transported on roads has increased by 30 per cent (Paxton 1994) and the average distance it has travelled has increased by nearly 60 per cent (Hoskins and Lobstein 1998). Not only is the same amount of food being transported further, but British consumers are also travelling further to get it. They use – almost have to use – cars to do so. The distance travelled for shopping in general rose by 60 per cent between 1975/6 and 1989/91, but the travel taken by car more than doubled (Raven *et al.* 1995). Far from hypermarkets being convenient, they in fact generate more, not less, trips for food shopping. UK Government figures also indicate that the mileage of trips to town-centre food shops is less than half that of trips taken to edge-of-town stores (Whitelegg 1994). The distance food travels within the food system before it is consumed illustrates the economic problem of externalities. The price of modern food systems does not reflect the true price of production.

The transition from rural to urban living

Worldwide there are now more people living in urban than rural areas. Farmers are generally leaving the land, while holdings concentrate. This applies even in rich areas of the world. The Organization for Economic Co-operation and Development (OECD) has noted falls in both farm and food processing employment between 1985 and 1994 (OECD 1998). In France, home of the small food entrepreneur, farm holdings have declined from 1 million to 680 000 in the last decade.

As the population in cities continues to expand into the twenty-first century, the demand for food to feed urban people will grow. The FAO estimates that in a city of 10 million people, 6000 tonnes of food may need to be imported on a daily basis (FAO 1998). By the year 2025, there will be a huge increase in the numbers of people in the south living in cities. Between 1950 and 1990, the world's towns and cities grew twice as fast as rural areas. In 1950, only two cities had more than 8 million inhabitants, London and New York (Harrison 1992). It is estimated that over the next 20 years, 93 per cent of urban growth will take place, whilst the majority of the population in the continents of Africa and Asia will remain in the rural areas. Many cities in the world already have huge populations. For example Dhaka in Bangladesh has a population of 9 million and is growing at an annual rate of 5 per cent, an extra 1300 people per day (FAO 1998). Asian cities are now growing at a rate of 3 per cent per year, while African cities are growing at a rate of 4 per cent per year.

In 2025, an estimated two out of three people in the world will live in urban areas. Fed by whom and on what? Traders argue that this makes them essential, but the question raised here is whether that trade should be local, regional, or global? The policy choice is not the old stark choice of free trade or protectionism/autarky, beloved of economic theoreticians, but of what sort of trade? The policy challenge is how to judge what could and should be produced locally rather than be transported round the globe.

One US neo-liberal policy position argues that China's affluence will lead to never-ending demand for meat which only overproducing-grain areas like the USA will be able to satiate. This discussion is barely tempered by a health dimension, when it ought to be, if only because Chinese data provides some of the best benchmarking for the connection between diet and health. The huge Chinese study referred to earlier also showed that the higher the fat intake, even within a relatively low fat-consuming culture, the greater the health impact (Chen *et al.* 1990).

Globally, the World Bank has estimated that there will be over one billion urban poor in the twenty-first century (World Bank 1997). In 1950, the number of people living in cities was about the same in industrialized and in developing countries – about 300 million (World Bank 1999). By 2000, some two billion people will live in cities in developing countries, more than twice the number of urban dwellers in industrialized countries. As populations in cities expand, so does the demand for food to feed all the people who are living there. Even allowing for urban food production – gardens, smallholdings, even window boxes – the majority of food in the city must be bought. Poor families can spend as much as 60–80 per cent of their income on food. People in cities spend approximately a third more on food than their rural neighbours. With this urbanization, the problem of food security grows.

At the Habitat 2 conference in Turkey in 1996, the UN Development Programme mapped out the urgency of the task. Its conclusion was that urban or peri-urban agriculture, far from being something from the past, will once more become important (UNDP 1996). In Kathmandu, 37 per cent of urban gardeners already grow all the vegetables they consume, while in Hong Kong, 45 per cent of demand for vegetables is supplied from 5–6 per cent of the land mass. Across the world, there is an interesting and hopeful movement of local authorities, small farmers, and ecology-conscious and confidence-seeking consumers arguing for, and supporting, this modern urban agriculture sector. The WHO European Region's Nutrition Programme, for instance, has argued that local produce can provide food security for otherwise marginalized populations (WHO–Europe 1998).

This is particularly relevant to eastern Europe which has witnessed catastrophic collapses in currencies. To import (expensive) foods, one needs a strong currency. Projects such as community gardens and city farms have also sprung up in the industrial heartlands, showing that urban food production has a social as well as economic value (Pretty 1998). Real market-economies offer some solutions for this potential disaster by encouraging local production to meet local need. What is 'local' is relative. If it is planned well, located in a place which people can easily access the food and is well organized and hygienic, urban agriculture can be a good source of income for urban workers and help boost the local economy (Garnett 1999). Experience suggests, however, that if urban agriculture is born out of necessity – such as happened in Russia, particularly in the economic turmoil after the collapse of communism –

rather than out of choice or conviction, the moment people have the option to purchase rather than grow some or all of their food, they often will. In this respect, the
policy challenge for the future is how to reinvigorate a food culture which sees the
positive benefits of urban agriculture (WHO–Europe 1998).

The economic transition

A key factor in analysing trade's impact on health must be not just *what* trade
does but *how* it does it. To begin to assess this, it is necessary to appreciate the main
features of the modern food economy. The reality is that health is somewhat marginal
as a driver. Food business interest in health is generally fairly narrowly limited to food
safety and that after numerous scandals around the world. Health controls have too
often been swept away in the name of trade liberalization when they really deserved to
be modernized and strengthened (London Food Commission 1988). Pressure from
consumer campaigns on safety, environmental, and ethical concerns are of course
now a factor in boardroom discussions. But the approach there is defensive rather
than proactive. A safety scandal is bad for a brand.

In main, the food sector – certainly in the west – is characterized by the following
features:

+ a rapid economic concentration in all food sectors, both through organic growth
  and mergers and acquisition within and across national borders

+ a fragmentation of markets and a seemingly endless pursuit of new niche markets

+ comparatively rapid, commercially driven changes in diet and taste

+ a ceaseless pursuit of quality control via supply chain management (Trienekens
  and Zuurbier 1996)

+ intensification both on and off the land, in order to raise yields of land, labour and
  capital

+ transformation of foods and food processes across sectors; not only have the
  nature of farming and storage been transformed but even cooking

+ the growth of size and influence of the distributors and retailers within the food
  system, representing a transition from producer to retail power

+ an ideological tension over the state's role, both over responsibilities for law
  enforcement and for education of the public about food matters

+ an unmanageability in the consumer body politic, with a growth of consumerism
  threatening predictability for dominant forces within the food system (Gabriel
  and Lang 1995)

+ promotion of brands as a response to consumer desire for certainty

+ ever more sophisticated use of the 'consciousness' industries, such as advertising,
  marketing, product placement and sponsorship, to increase brand value

+ new inequalities within and between countries creating modern forms of food
  poverty even in rich countries

♦ centralization of decision making nationally, regionally, and internationally, with tensions between all levels

♦ a pivotal battle for world markets between the EU and the USA which threatens to marginalize the interest of the rest of the world.

This economic situation is both driven by and threatening to food companies, yet the late twentieth century was a period of exploding corporate power in the food system. In the case of wheat, for instance, whereas in the past cereals would be grown, milled, cooked, and consumed locally, today a handful of companies dominate the world market (Morgan 1979). Whereas wheat originated in the middle east, it is today one of the most traded and travelled of food commodities, being grown worldwide wherever climate allows it.

One company, Cargill, now dominates the world cereals (not just wheat) market and has the power to buy major competitors. Mergers and acquisitions (M&As) are rife throughout the food chain to such an extent that they now trouble observers of competition, let alone health, policy (Krebs 1999). A wave of M&As has shrunk the number of key grain traders, for instance, from seven global giants in the 1970s to just four. Food corporations can use their purchasing, contracting, and specifications-setting power to exert considerable control throughout the food supply chain. Cargill, for instance, is the USA's largest animal feed plant owner, the fifth largest turkey producer, the fourth largest pork packer, the fifth largest ethanol producer, and so on (Heffernan 1999).

This power is not without exposure and dangers. Cargill had to write off huge sums when Russia defaulted on its debt in August 1998 (Corrigan 1999). The battle for domination of the world 'sweet tooth' market, for instance, is now between interests representing sugar cane, sugar beet, maize (isoglucose), and artificial sweeteners (for example aspartame). The new era is characterized by huge companies thinking about food just as the giant automobile companies can think about cars: locating design, production, and assembly in different parts of the world, and enabling flexible systems to emerge. Even so their huge investments can leave them exposed to currency fluctuations.

The scale on which huge corporations are able to think today dwarfs even the power of the giants of previous eras such as the East India Company which held sway over British India in the eighteenth and early nineteenth centuries. Using satellite mapping and computer-based data storage and planning, food companies today are able to organize the planting and distribution of crops more holistically and speedily than before (Thrupp 1995). Just-in-time supply chain management systems are essential for global reach. Studies of the international lettuce, strawberry, and vegetable markets, for instance, have shown how extensive this global reach can be and also how their routes have developed from farm to end consumer (Feder 1977; Friedland *et al.* 1981; Thrupp 1995). This modern, trans-national pattern of control has been unfolding for decades (George 1976) and is, to reiterate the central point, but another phase in the two centuries-old industrialization of agriculture. Sugar, for instance, has been produced in a global system for centuries, utilizing an international division of labour (Fine *et al.* 1996; Raynolds 1997).

The characteristics of modern global food business

The global reach of large food corporations is now a major 'driver' behind dietary change. It is also a major threat to national or local firms. In Vietnam, for instance, international branded ice cream is better funded and has the advantages of up-market foreign cachet, both expanding the market in dairy products (in a low dairy consuming country) and their market share (Birchall 1999). Such brand marketing is facilitated by revolutions in distribution and production within and between continents which large companies are well able to exploit. In 2000, Unilever, one of the largest food companies in the world, decided to rationalize its brand portfolio from 1600 to 400 key brands in order to promote them more effectively worldwide. Its strategic decision to do this lay behind its decision to sell of some smaller brands while purchasing for US$20.3 billion the US food giant Bestfoods, owner of existing world brands such as Hellman's mayonnaise and Knorr soups (Tomkins 2000). Having purchased these brands, to extract value it must now promote and extend them. Yet who is there to champion the health costs of changing food tastes that result?

Concentration of market share is a key feature of the modern food economy. Table 6.1 shows how the largest among existing giants are mainly North American or European (Rural Advancement Foundation International 1999), while Table 6.2 shows the level of concentration that can emerge when a market goes truly global, in this case agrichemicals (Agrow 1999). The top 10 agrochemical corporations account for US$26.2 billion or 85 per cent of the US$30.9 billion agrochemical market worldwide. Table 6.3 illustrates the high levels of concentration in agricultural inputs (Rural Advancement Foundation International 1999). The top 10 seed companies control

Table 6.1 The world's top ten food & beverage companies

Company	1997 Food & drink sales US $ millions	Food & drink as % of total revenues
Nestlé SA (Switzerland)	45,380	95%
Philip Morris Co. Inc. (USA)	31,890	44%
Unilever Plc/NV (UK & Netherlands)	24,170	50%
ConAgra, Inc. (USA)	24,000	100%
Cargill, Inc. (USA)	21,000	38%
PepsiCo, Inc. (USA)	20,910	100%
Coca-Cola Co. (USA)	18,860	100%
Diageo (UK) Guinness + GrandMetropolitan (UK)	18,770	93%
Mars Inc. (USA)	14,000	100%
Danone (France)	13,970	94%

Source: Rural Advancement Foundation International 1999, 4

Table 6.2 World top ten agrichemical companies, 1998 sales

Company	Country base	Sales (US $ millions)	% Change 1997–8
Novartis	Switzerland	$4,152	−1.1%
Monsanto	USA	$4,032	23%
DuPont	USA	$3,156	26%
Zeneca	UK	$2,897	8.3%
AgrEvo	Germany	$2,410	2.5%
Bayer	Germany	$2,273	0.2%
Rhone-Poulene	France	$2,266	2.9%
Cyanamid	USA	$2,194	3.5%
Dow Agro-Sci	USA	$2,132	11%
BASF	Germany	$1,945	4.9%

Source: Agrow, 1999

approximately 32 per cent of the US$23 billion seed trade worldwide. Even though an estimated two-thirds of all seeds sown annually are currently farmer grown, i.e. seeds kept back from a preceding crop rather than commercially purchased, this is a remarkable figure.

The move into genetic engineering represents an attempt to erode this farmer-derived market and to build in commercial dependency. Although consumer reaction is threatening this trend – not just through protest or product pressure but also legal anti-trust cases (Eaglesham 1999) – the rapid entry of genetically modified (GM) seeds in the home US market testifies to the effectiveness of this commercial strategy. Table 6.4 shows the rapid growth of GM crops in some major cereal exporting countries (Rural Advancement Foundation International 1999), but this is dwarfed by the USA. Based on the area planted in 1998, one company, Monsanto had 88 per cent of the US market, Aventis (AgrEvo) had 8 per cent, and Novartis had 4 per cent. In most national markets, this would be deemed a monopoly Rural Advancement Foundation International (1999).

Table 6.5 gives the top five baby food companies, by world sales (British Medical Association 1999). It is corporations like these that bodies such as the WHO and the United Nations Children's Fund (UNICEF) have to deal with when trying to implement the commitment to promote good neo-natal health through breast-feeding. Nestlé is both the largest food company and the largest baby food company in the world.

The transition from market to hypermarket economy

The classic conception of a market economy that underpins the dominant policy approach to trade imputes that its efficiencies are achieved when many sellers vie for the attention of many consumers. This is indeed the market relationship one can

Table 6.3 The world's top ten seed corporations

Company	1997 Revenue US $ millions	Comment
DuPont/Pioneer Hi-Bred International (USA)	$1,800+	DuPont owns 20% share in Pioneer DuPont will buy the remaining share of Pioneer for$7.7 billion
Monsanto (USA)	$1,800 (estimate)	Estimate of the total sales volume of all Monsanto seed acquisitions made by October, 1998 (66)
Novartis (Switzerland)	$928	Formerly Ciba Geigy and Sandoz
Groupe Limagrain (France)	$686	French co-operative
Advanta (UK and Netherlands)	$437	Owned by AstraZeneca and Royal VanderHave
AgriBiotech, Inc. (USA)	$425	The company has completed over 30 acquisitions (forage and turfgrass) since 1995
Grupo Pulsar/Seminis/ ELM (Mexico) has merged with Seguros Comerical America; the joint company is	$375	Pulsar is giant agro-industrial corporation that owns Empresas La Moderna, majority shareholder of Seminis, Inc.
Savia		
Sakata (Japan)	$349	Vegetable/flower/turfgrass
KWS AG (Germany)	$329	Major sugar-beet seed company
Takii (Japan)	$300 (estimate)	Privately-held

Source: Rural Advancement Foundation International 1999, 7

note in classic street markets, for instance in many developing countries, where local goods are offered to local consumers. In many developed market sectors and developed countries, however, a different relationship between production and consumption has emerged, in which the distributor not consumer is sovereign. The hypermarket economy has arrived. And with giant retailers such as the US Wal-Mart (now the ninth largest corporation in the world) (Financial Times 1999) expanding overseas from the USA to Canada, Mexico, Germany, and the UK, and with Royal Dutch Ahold expanding from north Europe to the USA, what might better be termed the food retail mega-market economy is emerging. Ahold, for instance, has purchased Giant stores in the USA for US$2.8 billion. Although only Europe's tenth largest food retailer, it has chains in the USA, Latin America, and South East Asia too. It has 40 stores in Shanghai alone (Hollinger 1998).

Table 6.4 Area of transgenic crops planted (millions of hectares)

Country	1997	1998
USA	8.1	20.5
Argentina	1.4	4.3
Canada	1.3	2.8
Australia	0.1	0.1
Mexico	0.1	0.1
Spain	0.0	0.1
France	0.0	0.1
South Africa	0.0	0.1
TOTAL	11.0	27.8

Source: Rural Advancement Foundation International 1999, 7

Wal-Mart already has 3400 stores on four continents and it has a global long-term strategy (Ortega 1998). 'Our priorities are that we want to dominate North America first, then South America, and then Asia and then Europe', the Chief Executive has said (Weissman 1999). Even in an area known for its dynamic small- and medium-sized enterprise (SME) sector like Hong Kong, two companies owned by conglomerates control an estimated 70 per cent of market share (Lucas 1999). The threat posed to such control by electronic shopping is more apparent than real, as companies financially as well resourced as these have the capacity to go on-line when others have pioneered the methodology.

It has been argued that these trends signify an important change in trade from that of a market economy to one of the hypermarket economy (Raven et al. 1995). In the hypermarket economy, supply chain management is the key. Retailers are sovereign because they mediate between production and consumption. A survey by USA-based Management Ventures, a consultancy which tracks retail spending in the world's 73 largest economies, found that between 1994 and 1999, the top 200 retailers (all retailing not just food) increased their share of retail spending from 21 to 28 per cent, and estimated that this would rise to 50 per cent by the year 2009. The study estimated that the top 25 will then have annual sales of US$140 billion, a figure today only reached by the world's biggest retailer, Wal-Mart of the USA (Hollinger 1999a). When two huge French retailers Carrefour and Promodes merged in 1999, they created the second largest food retailer in the world with stores in 26 countries; the new group became overnight the biggest retailer in France, Spain, Belgium, Portugal, Greece, Brazil, Argentina, Taiwan, and Indonesia.

Carrefour's chairman has spelled out a clear vision: 'We will have local companies or global companies but not much in between. Globalisation will lead those that are not in the first team, or who are national retailers, to make alliances' (Hollinger 1999b). He saw three forces pushing the top retailers to further globalization: firstly the growing sophistication of consumers pressurizing the retailer (Gabriel and Lang

Table 6.5 Top five global baby food companies, by turnover

Company	Employees	Head office	Founded	Main business	Countries of operation	Turnover
Nestlé SA	231,881	Switzerland	1867	Beverages, milk products, nutrition and ice cream	Nestle has over 500 factories in more than 80 countries	US $52 billion (1998)
SMA/Wyeth/AHP	52,984	USA	1860	AHP: health care and crop protection	AHP: 'more than 100'	AHP:US $13.5 billion (1998)
Abbott-Ross	56,236	USA	1900	Nutrition, pharmaceuticals, health care and agricultural products	'more than 130 world-wide'	US $12.5 billion (1998)
Mead-Johnson/ Bristol-Myers Squibb	54,700	USA	1856 (Squibb)	Pharmaceuticals, consumer medicines, beauty care, nutritional and medical devices	BMS: 'more than 100 countries'	BMS: US $18 billion (1998)
Numico	10,577	Netherlands	1896	Nutritional products	In 50 countries	US $1.85 billion (1998)

Source: Baby Milk Action (British Medical Association, 1999)

Table 6.6 The world's top ten food retailers, by sales 1998

Rank	Company	Parent country	Sales, US $ billions
1	Wal-Mart	USA	123.2
2	Metro	Germany	49.0
3	Kroger	USA	38.6
4	Intermarché	France	36.6
5	Ahold	Netherlands	34.9
6	Carrefour*	France	33.8
7	Auchan	France	23.6
8	Leclerc	France	23.1
9	Promodes*	France	20.6
10	Casino	France	14.8

Source: Financial Times (Iskander 1999)
Note: *merged 1999 to create the new global no.2

1995), secondly, capital intensification and thirdly, the need 'to extract the best price from their suppliers to be able to stay competitive.' Table 6.6 gives the world's top 10 food retailers by sales in 1998 (Iskander 1999).

The transition from supermarket to mega-market has considerable direct and indirect health implications. An immediate effect has been closure of small shops, meaning that consumers have to go further to stores when they just want a few goods (Ritzer 1999); car use increases, physical exercise in daily life drops. With obesity levels rising alarmingly across the world (obesity is a risk factor for heart disease) (WHO 1998), and in some respects one of the world's most significant health trends, it is absurd that people burn fossil fuels rather than food as fuel. It is absurd that people then go to gyms to take exercise in safety – often on walking or running machines! – rather than burn off food energy in their daily lives. The healthy solution is surely to build exercise into daily life.

Another impact is on employment. With the world already highly fragmented into high earners and low/no earners (over a billion people survive on less that a US$ a day), hypermarketization symbolizes the macro-economic question of quality of work. Is the emergence of more part-time, casual, and low status work associated with 'McDonaldization' a societal bonus or drain? Is total employment created or reduced? Companies claim that new jobs are created. They undoubtedly are but critics dispute the overall gain, pointing to lost jobs in smaller stores. In the UK, a report by the National Retail Planning Forum in 1998 examined the effect on jobs in food retailing within a 10 mile radius over a four-year period following the opening of 93 edge-of-town superstores. Taking into account all the new jobs provide by the superstores, there was a net average loss of 276 jobs per store, making a national total loss of 25 000 jobs in that period (Fell 1999; Porter and Raistrick 1998).

Challenges for public health

If the analysis above is correct, an awesome set of challenges faces health professionals and others involved in the development of health policy.

What then, should health-policy makers contribute to food and trade policy? They face choices of direction. In one direction lie further intensification of food and farming systems and further externalization of financial, environmental, and social costs, whilst in another direction lies a more sustainable, lower technology vision for food and farming. Both scenarios offer risks, some known and others less well documented. Most investment over the last half century has favoured the former vision but there is increasing support for the latter vision both from civil society and more importantly from central and international governments and agencies. However, at present investment is still hopelessly unequal and too often health, environmental, or community concerns are treated as 'bolt-on extras' rather than intrinsic values. The central and immediate challenge for health-policy makers is to ensure that they are better informed about the entire food system. The goal ought to be for evidence-based policies. It is also in the interests of health-policy makers not to collude with a view which ultimately marginalizes them. This is why food governance needs to be improved and made more sensitive. If health is inadequately subsumed to corporate interests, health loses.

Governance and public health: the case for urgency

Food provides both a warning on, and an excellent illustration of, the complexity of the relationship between trade and society, human, and environmental health. Since its binding commitments to food as a right in 1948, the UN system has delivered a steady stream of important conferences, commissions and expert reports but all with non-binding legal status. The 1974 World Food Conference, the 1992 International Conference on Nutrition and the 1996 World Food Summit (WHO/FAO 1992) all produced excellent but non-binding plans of action. In 1992, the Earth Summit in Rio produced stronger environmental commitments. Yet by 2000, the FAO concluded that many of the goals set at the 1992 Earth Summit in Rio de Janeiro had still not been met. One of the goals was to help developing countries use resources more efficiently through sustainable agriculture and rural development programs. However, the FAO says most such efforts are still getting off the ground, while land degradation, loss of agro-biodiversity, and climate change continue apace.

Progress in reducing hunger (let alone tackling the diet-related degenerative diseases), according to the FAO, has been slow. In developing countries, 790 million people and elsewhere, 34 million suffer from hunger and malnourishment. The 1996 World Food Summit, hosted in Rome, had set a target of reducing those numbers by 20 million per year. However, since 1996, the number of hungry people has fallen by only eight million per year (UN Commission on Sustainable Development 2000). By 2000, the FAO Report on the State of World Food Security concluded that all these non-binding targets to reduce malnutrition – at its extreme still the most shocking diet and health issue – could not be achieved.

Is this a failure of public policy or practice? For centuries – particularly since the Irish Famine in the mid-nineteenth century – there has been a steady strand of critics of the role of trade, if left unfettered. As Nobel Prize-winner Amartya Sen, among others, have shown, hunger follows poor purchasing power and is not necessarily a function of food availability (Sen 1997, 1981, 2000). Throughout the twentieth century, attempts were made to soften liberal economics. Welfare safety nets were instituted in a piecemeal way by governments and after World War 2, a governmental responsibility to ensure all its people were adequately fed was technically enshrined in the Declaration of Human Rights. But after a few decades in which Keynesian economics was the orthodoxy, neo-liberal economics resumed pre-eminence (Cockett 1994). Why does this matter for public health?

Firstly, the institutions through which a public health perspective was mediated throughout the post-World War 2 period, namely the UN system of the WHO, FAO, and UNICEF, have gradually been marginalized. The new system of world trade governance under the WTO, but also with other trade-oriented institutional legacies such as the G7 and OECD, is now more powerful than the UN bodies (Banerji 1999; Navarro 1999). Both WTO and UN bodies are technically democratically answerable to governments but in practice, the UN bodies have more well-established systems of accountability and responsiveness to civic society. There is a World Health Assembly with the WHO but no parallel citizen's voice for the WTO. Hence the opposition at Seattle in 1999. Under the GATT Agreement on Agriculture, for example, national governments cannot set food standards or restrict entry of foods unless they have 'sound scientific' justification. This seems reasonable, but in practice – witness the issues of antibiotics, hormones, dioxin residues – the science is at best never entirely clear and at worst warped by commercially confidential studies.

Under the Technical Barriers to Trade (TBT) and Sanitary and Phytosanitary Standards (SPS) agreements of the GATT, arbitration on scientific standards gave 'influence' to the UN Codex Alimentarius Commission. Alas, this older body was not in a fit democratic state to accept this onerous responsibility. Too often, companies are present at Codex meetings where their products' safety is being evaluated (Avery *et al.* 1993). When just ten companies control 85 per cent of the US$31 billion annual world pesticides market (UNDP 1999), their power and presence at such meetings should not be underestimated (and is another reason an alliance representing public health, welding professions, institutions, NGOs, and citizenship interests is urgently needed at these GATT talks) (Labonte 1998). A study of the SPS on hormones and avocado pests concluded that using 'sound science' is 'a slippery objective' (Powell 1997). In practice, it is hard to separate political considerations or research funding from science.

The role of science in the arbitration/adjudication on food trade disputes is now particularly sensitive. For the last few years there has been a steady stream of high-profile cases where food exporting nations fight over the right to export surpluses to each other and to markets they deem their own. There have been wars over lamb between Australia, New Zealand, and the USA (International Centre for Trade and Sustainable Development 1999); over beef hormones between the EU and USA; over GM foods between the USA and many countries but especially the EU. Some of these trade disputes receive mass media coverage; others are covered in the specialist press only. They deserve open public health scrutiny. A main reason for this is that despite many intergovernmental commitments to allow, even encourage, nation states to ensure food security for their people (WHO/FAO 1992), the notion that food security stems from growing most of one's food within one's country (what used to be called self-reliance) is being replaced by the notion that security stems from being able to purchase food on the open world markets (WHO–Europe 1995). Experience from sub-Saharan Africa suggests that this is a policy for affluent countries rather than poor ones. If your exports are primary commodities and these are declining in worth, you have to export more just to stand still, let alone import basic food needs. As a policy it is folly.

While food security is a concern for most developing country governments, rich countries have been troubled by consumer-driven food safety issues. As the WHO Regional Office for Europe's Food and Nutrition Plan recognizes (WHO–Europe 1999), from a public health perspective, both are important and both reflect changes in methods of production and distribution and in the food system (Lang 1997; Tansey and Worsley 1995). In a paper prepared in June 1999, Norway laid down a clear policy challenge: food security is too important to be left to the vagaries of trade (Royal Ministry of Agriculture 1999). Under the plan of action agreed at the 1996 World Food Summit, as at the earlier 1992 International Conference on Nutrition, governments agreed that they have a moral responsibility to ensure their citizens have adequate food, are free from hunger, and achieve food security (World Food Summit 1996). The thorny issue is which is the best way to achieve it: grow your own or buy in? This question is now serious politics in India, for instance, where hundreds of thousands of farmers are resisting attempts to introduce genetically engineered seeds from US companies.

At its most unfettered, the pro-trade perspective favours the market approach to food security. Tacitly, it argues that the cheapest food is best. This chapter has proposed that the future lies with a new or ecological public health perspective. According to this, the West's twentieth-century food revolution-intensified food production successfully cheapened food but by externalizing other costs (Lang 1999c). This is the legacy which the twenty-first century has to grapple with. Far-sighted governments now realise this. Sweden, for instance, has set out to reduce its energy use, increase its biodiversity, and meet public health goals for its food sector (Environment Agency and Ministry of Agriculture 2000). Norway has also staked out an intellectual position in which trade rules should safeguard national food security. When wheat or maize prices can rise by 50 per cent in just two years, as happened in 1993–95, reliance on being able to buy one's food in the world market place is a form of security only open to the affluent. Norway, as a small population with immense oil wealth is ironically one such country.

The WTO structures are designed to facilitate cross-border economic activity and to reduce national control over capital flows, competition, and even cultural control. In the age of the Internet, information knows few boundaries yet vast new corporations are emerging which dominate almost everything humans do or consume. The irony about the 1994 GATT and its key Agreement on Agriculture is that they were based on the free trade model of globalization just when evidence about its negative effects was mounting up. According to the tenth annual UN Human Development

Report, the richest 20 per cent of the world now account for 86 per cent of world Gross Domestic Product (GDP), while the poorest 20 per cent have just 1 per cent (UNDP 1999). Two hundred of the world's richest people have doubled their net worth in the last four years. The richest three people in the world have assets greater than the combined Gross National Product of all the least developed countries in the world, 600 million people. There is little chance of health for all in such a socially divided world.

The Human Development Report itself came into existence because in the late 1980s, UN administrators, social scientists, and politicians were critical of the convention of measuring development through indicators such as Gross Domestic or National Product. They disguise intranational inequalities and fail to convey the quality-of-life issues. The Human Development Index was created to fill this gap. The Human Development Report shows that 80 countries have incomes lower today than a decade ago. Over a fifth of humanity (1.3 billion people), exist on less than US$1 per day. However it is measured, the gap between the richest and poorest is widening. In 1960, the gap between the richest fifth and the poorest fifth was 30:1. In 1990 it was 60:1. In 1997 it was 74:1 (UNDP 1999). In this context, it is clear that epidemiologists as much as physicians and health activists have to ask themselves how their work does or does not confront this obscene accrual of wealth and power. The issue is no longer whether we are for or against trade but who gains from it, and what sort of trade it is.

The Human Development Report argued that globalization is unstoppable and that all good people can do is try to give it 'development with a human face'. This chapter has suggested that, on the contrary, the public health challenge is not more globalization but how to rebuild local production everywhere to enable just trade and food security. The good news is that proponents of unfettered free trade are more defensive since Seattle (Wolf 1999). Inequalities may be bad, they admit, but now is the time to target resources on the poor. We should ignore, they imply, the accrual of power by the rich as they are the motor force of the new global economy. This argument is seductive but bad public health. We know that less divided countries have better public health (Wilkinson 1996). So why argue for the 'trickle down' theory by another name?

There may be good historical grounds for trying to ameliorate the worst excesses of globalization, as the Human Development Report suggests. But we should also recognize that many public health gains have been won when the affluent and the middle classes recognize that they cannot escape socially induced ill health among the poor and that it is in their interests to tackle the causes of ill health together. Confronting vested interest may actually be the best chance we have of putting the 'human face' on globalization. The trade sector and the WTO/GATT talks are very serious politics; noone listens to arguments unless they come to the table with clout. The negotiations are raw geo-politics. The challenge for public health generally, and certainly in food policy, is to argue hard and fast for a tough proactive health perspective. Getting the odd sentence in a 2000-page agreement will not suffice. If trade agreements diminish the room for proactive health intervention, we will only have ourselves to blame. The challenge now is to ensure that public health is fairly represented. If the WTO and accompanying ideology marginalize health, will national health ministries and the WHO confront them?

References

Adshead, S. A. M. (1992) *Salt and civilization.* Macmillan, London.

Agrow (1999) *World Crop Protection News*, March 26 and April 16.

Alexandros, N. (1995) *World agriculture: towards 2010.* Wiley, Chichester/FAO, Rome.

Avery, N., Drake, M., and Lang, T. (1993) *Cracking the codex.* National Food Alliance, London.

Banerji, D. A. (1999) A fundamental shift in the approach to international health by WHO, UNICEF, and the World Bank: instances of the practices of "intellectual facism" and the totalitarianism in some Asian countries. *International Journal of Health Services,* **29**(2), 227–59.

Barker, D. J. P. (ed.) (1992) *Fetal and infant origins of adult disease.* British Medical Journal Books, London.

Barnet, R. and Cavanagh, J. (1994) *Global dreams: imperial corporations and the new world order.* Simon and Schuster, New York.

Bianchini, F., Corbetta, F., and Pistoia, M. (1988) *The fruits of the earth.* Bloomsbury, London.

Birchall, J. (1999) Foreign groups fuel ice cream wars in Vietnam. *Financial Times*, January 5.

British Medical Association (1999) *Baby milk action up-date.* British Medical Association, London.

Brown, L. R., Renner, M., and Halweil, B. (1999) *Vital signs.* W W Norton, New York/Earthscan, London.

Cannon, G. (1992) Food and health: the experts agree: an analysis of one hundred authoritative scientific reports on food, nutrition and public health published throughout the world in thirty years between 1961 and 1991. Consumers' Association, London.

Castells, M. (1996) *The information age: economy, society and culture.* Oxford: Blackwell.

Chen, J., Campbell, T. C., Li, J., and Peto, R. (1990) *Diet, lifestyle and mortality in China: A Study of the Characteristics of 65 Countries.* Oxford University Press, Oxford.

Cockett, R. (1994) *Thinking the Unthinkable: Think-tanks and the economic counter-revolution 1931–1983.* Harper Collins, Oxford.

Commission on the Nutrition Challenges of the 21st Century (2000) Ending malnutrition by 2020: an agenda for change in the millennium: final report to the ACC/SCN. Administrative Committee on Co-ordination, Sub-Committee on Nutrition (ACC/SCN) of the United Nations, New York.

Corrigan, T. (1999) Cargill operating earnings tumble by 53%. *Financial Times*, August 12, p. 20.

Dalby, A. (1996) *Siren feasts: a history of food and gastronomy in Greece.* Routledge, London.

Drewnoski, A. and Popkin, B. (1997) The nutrition transition: new trends in the global diet, *Nutrition Reviews*, **55**, 31–43.

Eaglesham, J. (1999) Antitrust case sows seeds of debate about farming future. *Financial Times*, September 13.

Environment Agency and Ministry of Agriculture (2000) The 2021 initiatives of the Environment Agency and Ministry of Agriculture, Stockholm

FAO (1998) *The state of food and agriculture.* FAO, Rome.

FAO (1999) *The state of food insecurity in the world.* FAO, Rome.

Feder, E. (1977) *Strawberry imperialism.* Institute of Social Studies, Den Haag, Netherlands.

Fell, D. (1999) The impact of out-of-centre food superstores on local retail employment. National Retailing Planning Forum Occasional Paper Series 3, London.

Financial Times (1999) FT 500: Annual survey. *Financial Times*, January 28.

Fine, B., Heasman, M., and Wright, J. (1996) *Consumption in the age of affluence: the world of food.* Routledge, London.

Friedland, W., A, B. and Thomas, R. (1981) *Manufacturing green gold: capital, labour and technology in the lettuce industry.* Cambridge University Press, Cambridge.

Gabriel, Y. and Lang, T. (1995) *The unmanageable consumer.* Sage, London.

Gallup (1995) Financial Times Exporter. *Financial Times.*

Garnett, T. (1999) City harvest: the feasibility of growing more food in London. Sustain, London.

Geissler, C. (1999) China: the soybean-pork dilemma. *Proceedings of the Nutrition Society,* **58**, 345–53.

George, S. (1976) *How the other half dies.* Penguin, Harmondsworth.

Harrison, P. (1992) *The third revolution: environment, population and a sustainable world.* I B Tauris, New York.

Heffernan, W. (1999) Consolidation in the food and agriculture system. Report to the National Farmers Union (USA). University of Missouri Department of Rural Sociology, Missouri, Columbia.

Hobhouse, H. (1985) *Seeds of change: five plants that transformed mankind.* Sidgwick and Jackson, London

Hollinger, P. (1998) Shopping around for global status. *Financial Times,* November 20.

Hollinger, P. (1999a) Supermarkets go shopping for a merger. *Financial Times,* September 4.

Hollinger, P. (1999b) 'Carrefour's revolutionary'. *Financial Times,* December 4.

Hoskins, R. and Lobstein, T. (1998) *The pear essentials.* Sustainable Agriculture, Food and Environment Alliance, London.

International Centre for Trade and Sustainable Development (1999) Australia, New Zealand cry fowl over US lamb decision. *Bridges Weekly Trade News Digest,* **3**(27).

Iskander, S. (1999) Retailers plan biggest store chain in Europe. *Financial Times,* August 3.

Kim, J. Y., Millen, J. V., Irwin, A. *et al.* (2000) *Dying for growth: global inequality and the health of the poor.* Common Courage Press, Monroe, Maine.

Koivusalo, M. (1999) World Trade Organisation and trade-creep in health and social policies. GASPP Occasional Papers 4/1999. STAKES (National Research and Development Centre for Welfare and Health), Helsinki/Globalism and Social Policy Programme based at STAKES and Sheffield.

Krebs, A. (1999) Cargill's brazen effort to own US grain trade. *Agribusiness Examiner,* **45**(29 August).

Labonte, R. (1998) Healthy public policy and the World Trade Organisation: a proposal for an international health presence in future world trade/investment talks. *Health Promotion International,* **13**(3), 245–56.

Lambert, C. D. (1999) Testimony of National Cattlemen's Beef Association before the Subcommittee of the House Committee on Ways and Means: hearings on the United States negotiating objectives fo the WTO Seattle Ministerial Meeting. August 5.

Lang, T. (1992) Food fit for the world? How the GATT food trade talks challenge public health, the environment and the citizen. SAFE Alliance, London/ Public Health Alliance, Birmingham.

Lang, T. (1997) The public health impact of globalisation of food trade. In *Diet, nutrition and chronic disease: lessons from contrasting worlds,* ed. P. Shetty and K. McPherson, pp. 173–186. Wiley, London.

Lang, T. (1999a) The new GATT round: whose development? Whose health? *Journal of Epidemiology and Community Heath*, **53**, 681–2.

Lang, T. (1999b) The complexities of globalization: the UK as a case study of tensions within the food system and the challenge to food policy. *Agriculture and Human Values*, **16**, 169–85.

Lang, T. (1999c) Food as a public health issue. In *Perspectives in public health*, ed. S. Griffiths and H. D., pp. 47–58. Radcliffe Medical Press, Oxford.

London Food Commission (1988) *Food adulteration and how to beat it.* Unwin Hyman, London.

Lucas, L. (1999) Online supermarket forces big rivals to check out prices. *Financial Times*, August 9.

Marmot, M. Wilkinson, R. G. (eds) (1998) *The social determinants of health.* WHO Regional Office for Europe, Copenhagen.

Mintz, S. W. (1985) *Sweetness and power: the place of sugar in modern history.* Viking, New York.

Mintz, S. W. (1996) *Tasting food, tasting freedom: excursions into eating, culture and the past.* Beacon Press, Boston.

Morgan, D. (1979) *Merchants of grain.* Weidenfeld and Nicolson, London.

Murray, C. J. L. and Lopez, A. D. (1997) Mortality by cause for eight regions of the world: global burden of disease study. *The Lancet*, **349**(May), 1269–76, 347–52, 1436–42, 1498–1504.

Navarro, V. (1999) Health and equity in the world in the era of "globalisation". *International Journal of Health Services*, **29**(2), 215–26.

Norberg-Hodge, H. (1991) *Ancient futures: learning from Ladakh.* Sierra Club Books, San Francisco.

OECD (1998) Agricultural policy reform: stocktaking of achievements. Discussion Paper prepared for ECD Agriculture Committee, 506 March 1998. Organisation for Economic Co-operation and Development, Paris.

Ortega, B. (1998) In Sam we trust: the untold story of Sam Walton and how Wal-Mart is devouring America. Times Business, New York.

Paxton, A. (1994) The food miles report. SAFE Alliance, London.

Popkin, B. M. (1994) The nutrition transition in low-income countries: an emerging crisis. *Nutrition Reviews*, **52**, 285–98.

Porter, S. and Raistrick, P. (1998) *The impact of out-of-centre food superstores on local retail employment.* National Retailing Planning Forum Occasional Paper Series 2, London.

Powell, M. (1997) Science in sanitary and phytosanitary dispute resolution. Discussion Paper 97–50. Resources for the Future, Washington DC.

Pretty, J. (1998) *The living land.* Earthscan. London.

Raven, H., Lang, T., and Dumonteil, C. (1995) *Off our trolleys? food retailing and the hypermarket economy.* Institute for Public Policy Research, London.

Raynolds, L. (1997) Restructuring national agriculture, agro-food trade, and agrarian livelihoods in the Caribbean. In *Globalising food: agrarian questions and global restructuring*, ed. D. Goodman and M. Wats. Routledge, London.

Ritzer, G. (1997) *The Mcdonaldization Thesis.* Sage, London.

Ritzer, G. (1999) *Enchanting a disenchanted world: revolutionizing the means of consumption.* Pine Forge Press, Thousand Oaks, California.

Rosegrant, M. W., Leach, N., and Gerpacio, R. V. (1999) Alternative futures for world cereal and meat consumption. *Proceedings of the Nutrition Society*, **58**, 219–34.

Rowling, N. (1987) *Commodities: how the world was taken to market.* Free Association Books, London.

Royal Ministry of Agriculture (1999) *Food security and the role of domestic agricultural food production.* Royal Ministry of Agriculture, Oslo.

Rural Advancement Foundation International (1999) The gene giants, masters of the universe, www.rafi.org/communique/fltxt/19992.html.

Sanders, T. A. B. (1999) The nutritional adequacy of plant-based diets. *Proceedings of the Nutrition Society*, **58**, 265–9.

Sanderson, S. (1986) The emergence of the 'world steer': internationalisation and Foreign Domination in Latin American cattle production. In *Food, The State and International Political Economy: Dilemmas of Developing Countries*, ed. F. Tullis and W. Hollist. University of Nebraska Press, Lincoln NE, pp. 102–129.

Scholte, J. A. (2000) *Globalization: a critical introduction.* Macmillan, Basingstoke.

Sen, A. (**1981**) *Poverty and famines: an essay on entitlement and deprivation.* Clarendon Press, Oxford.

Sen, A. (**1997**) *Inequality re-Examined.* Oxford University Press, Oxford.

Sen, A. (**2000**) *Development and freedom.* Oxford University Press, Oxford.

Sen, A. and Dreze, J. (1981) Poverty and famines: an essay on entitlement and deprivation. International Labour Organisation, Geneva.

Smith, B. D. (1995) *The emergence of agriculture.* Scientific American Library, New York.

Tansey, G. and Worsley, T. (1995) *The food system.* Earthscan, London.

Taylor, A. and Thomas, C. (1999) *Global trade and global social issues.* Routledge, London.

Thrupp, L. A. (1995) *Bittersweet harvests for global supermarkets.* World Resources Institute, Washington DC.

Thruss, L. A. (1995) *Bittersweet harvests for global supermarkets: challenges in Latin America's agricultural export boom.* World Resources Institute, New York.

Tomkins, R. (2000) Manufacturers strike back. *Financial Times*, June 16.

Trienekens, E. G. and Zuurbier, P. J. P. (1996) *Proceedings of the 2nd International Conference on Chain Management in Agri-and Food Business.* Department of Management Studies, Wageningen Agricultureal University, The Netherlands.

UN Commission on Sustainable Development (2000) Press release, 20th April, http://www.unfoundation.org.

UNDP (1996) Urban agriculture: food, jobs and sustainable cities. Publication series for Habitat 2, Vol. 1. UNDP, New York.

UNDP (1999) Human development report. UNDP, New York.

Verster, A. (1996) Nutrition in transition: the case of the Eastern Mediterranean Region. In *Nutrition and Quality of Life: Health Issues for the 21st Century*, ed. P. Pietinen, C. Nishida, and N. Khaltaev. WHO, Geneva.

Weissman, R. (1999) Wal-Mart *Corporate Focus*, 9 November.

Whitelegg, J. (1994) *Driven to sheop.* Eco-Logica/Sustainable Agriculture, Food and Environmental Alliance, London.

WHO (1990) Diet, nutrition and the prevention of chronic diseases. Technical Report Series 797. WHO, Geneva.

WHO (1998) Obesity: preventing and managing the global epidemic. Report of a WHO consultation on obesity, WHO/NUT/NCD/98.1. WHO, Geneva.

WHO (1999) World health report 1999: making a difference. WHO, Geneva.

WHO–Europe (1995) Nutrition policy in WHO European member states. Progress report following the 1992 International Conference on Nutrition. WHO–Europe, Copenhagen.

WHO–Europe (1998) Draft urban food and nutrition action plan: elements for local action or local production for local consumption. WHO Regional Office for Europe programme for nutrition policy, infant feeding and food security, Copenhagen/ETC urban agriculture programme, Leusden, The Netherlands/WHO Centre for Urban Health.

WHO–Europe (1999) Draft food and nutrition action plan. WHO–Europe, Copenhagen.

WHO/FAO (1992) World declaration and plan of action for nutrition. *FAO/WHO International Conference on Nutrition.* FAO/WHO, Rome.

Wilkinson, R. G. (1996) *Unhealthy societies.* Routledge, London.

Winson, A. (1993) *The intimate commodity: food and the development of the agro-industrial complex in Canada.* Garamond Press, Toronto.

Wolf, M. (1999) A world divided. *Financial Times,* July 14.

World Bank (1997) *The global burden of disease.* World Bank, Washington DC

World Bank (1999) World development report 1999–2000. World Bank, Washington,

World Food Summit (1996) Objective 7.4. FAO, Rome.

Worldwatch Institute (2000) *State of the world 2000.* Norton, New York.

Chapter 7

War: from humanitarian relief to prevention

Douglas Holdstock

Introduction

War is bad for health: any land-mine victim or war widow will confirm this. It is, though, impossible to give accurate figures for the morbidity and mortality of war. Civilian deaths associated with war may be directly weapons related ('collateral' in today's jargon), or due to starvation or disease which would not otherwise have occurred, and estimates for different times and conflicts are not comparable in these respects. Allowing for this, there have been about 142 million war-related deaths (approximately 76 million military and 64 million civilian) between AD 1500 and 1990 (Sivard 1991), and 110 million (62 million civilian and 44 million military) from 1900–1995 (Sivard 1996); over 20 million have died in war *since* the end of World War 2. Even allowing for the population explosion of the twentieth century, the century just ended has clearly been one of war and violence, while at its end the technology of war – 'conventional' weapons as well as weapons of mass destruction – threatens far worse for the next. The prevention of war is therefore essential.

Military surgeons and nurses have always been integral members of the armed forces. Formal humanitarian relief in war began with Jean-Henri Dunant's formation of the Red Cross in 1863. Individual doctors opposed to war in principle made their views known from the nineteenth century onwards, and others have examined the psychological factors underlying war (Lewer 1992). In the twentieth century, organized physicians' movements providing humanitarian aid in war zones, or calling for the outlawing of specific weapon systems, or limitation or ending of all war, have multiplied.

Effective action to ameliorate the impact on health of the issues considered in this book requires political action. Such action will be opposed by various vested interests, as will any radical attempts to abolish war. The arms industry and its associated trade is second only in size to the oil industry, with obvious implications for employment, but war is an institution (Groebel and Hinde 1989; Hinde and Watson 1995). For Karl von Clausewitz (1780–1831) 'war [was] nothing more than the continuation of politics by other means'. With the increasing destructiveness of modern war, this attitude is becoming less overt, but still underlies the rhetoric of humanitarian intervention such as official justification of the recent wars in former Yugoslavia. Effective medical prevention of war will thus require co-operation between medical and other anti-war groups, aid, development and economic agencies, and sympathetic political movements.

In what follows, the health impact and response to specific types of weapons is first considered, followed by an examination of the role of the arms trade and a brief discussion of the broader political changes needed for a war-free – that is, stable – global society. For reasons of space, only a selected reference list is given, though, where possible, references with full citations of other work have been chosen. A fuller discussion of the impact of conflict on today's world can be found in the report of the Carnegie Commission (Carnegie Commission on Preventing Deadly Conflict 1992), and war as a public health issue is treated in depth by Sidel and Levy (Sidel and Levy 1997).

Nuclear weapons

The effect of nuclear weapons

Nuclear weapons are uniquely destructive. The bombs dropped on Hiroshima and Nagasaki killed well over 200 000 outright, or from injuries and radiation sickness over the next few months, with many more in later years; the incidence of some cancers in survivors is still greater than in comparable Japanese cities. Yet these were low-yield fission weapons, of yield 12 000–20 000 tons (12–20 kt), compared with 100 kt to a megaton or more for today's thermonuclear ('hydrogen') or fusion bombs. At the height of the Cold War, stockpiles, mainly in the USA and the Soviet Union, contained at least 70 000 warheads, and about 35 000 remain operational or in reserve at the beginning of the twenty-first century. Any one of these could wipe out a medium-sized city and the death and destruction that would amount from a major nuclear exchange was, and is, incalculable. Various reports have attempted to predict the effects of such an exchange, and stressed the impossibility of any sort of response by health care services, no matter how well prepared (British Medical Association Board of Science and Education 1983; Physicians for Social Responsibility 1962; World Health Organization (WHO) Management Group 1987, 1983). Warnings have been given that the smoke and dust thrown into the atmosphere would cause widespread climatic changes ('nuclear winter') with serious effects on the environment and agriculture, perhaps leading to global starvation (Harwell and Hutchinson 1985; Pittock *et al.* 1985). Today, several thousand nuclear weapons remain on high alert, and human or computer error could still lead to catastrophe (Forrow *et al.* 1998), both human and environmental.

The nuclear cycle

The industry producing these weapons may also have persistent health consequences, as could the civil nuclear power industry that developed from the reactors producing plutonium for nuclear weapons. Several thousand atmospheric nuclear tests produced radioactive fall-out, and standards of radiation protection in nuclear installations in the USA and Russia have often been poor. Radiation is a known carcinogen, and elevated cancer rates have recently been reported at 14 American nuclear weapons plants. Clusters of childhood leukaemia and lymphoma have been detected around the Sellafield reprocessing plant in Cumbria and the Atomic Weapons Establishment plant at Aldermaston in the UK. According to conventional models of radiation biology, exposures due to emissions from these plants are too small to cause such clusters, but safety standards at both have been criticized, and recent studies of the effects of alpha emitters such as plutonium question the reliability of the models (Wright 2000).

Eliminating nuclear weapons

Work towards a nuclear-weapon-free world is political. But accurate information about the health consequences of the nuclear cycle and of the effects of nuclear war, with the impossibility of any useful medical response to the latter, has already contributed to what progress there has been so far towards nuclear disarmament.

Increasing anxiety over radioactive fallout from nuclear weapon tests in the 1950s, and in particular over the bone-seeking strontium–90 as a potential cause of childhood leukaemia, led to the 1963 Partial Test Ban Treaty banning above-ground tests (for key multi-lateral treaties see Table 7.1.) In the USA., a group of Boston physicians founded Physicians for Social Responsibility to draw attention to the effects of thermonuclear weapons (Physicians for Social Responsibility 1962). With detente and below-ground tests, concern switched to the Vietnam war and human rights issues, but the nuclear issue resurfaced in the late 1970s with the advent of hawkish governments in the USA and UK, and the Soviet invasion of Afghanistan. The introduction of multiple-warhead missiles under satellite guidance led to talk of 'first-strike' and 'prevailing' in nuclear war. Official medical organizations such as the British Medical Association (British Medical Association Board of Science and Education 1983) and the WHO (WHO Management Group 1983, 1987) and unofficial groups in many countries expressed concern about these developments; many of the latter joined together to form International Physicians for Prevention of Nuclear War (IPPNW) in 1980 (for information on selected organizations see Table 7.2.) From the start, IPPNW saw its main role, representing physicians with bonds transcending national boundaries, in resisting the increasing east–west split underlying the nuclear stand-off of the 1980s, and this was a major factor in its receiving the Nobel Peace Prize in 1985. As part of the worldwide peace movement, making use of modern electronic communications, medical groups continue to press for a nuclear-weapon-free world.

The International Court of Justice opinion

The World Court Project, a network of international non-governmental organizations (NGOs) including IPPNW, helped to obtain an advisory opinion from the UN's principal judiciary body, the International Court of Justice (ICJ) on 'the legality of the threat of use of nuclear weapons'. The WHO reports (WHO Management Group 1983, 1987) were a principal source of evidence to the court. In its opinion (International Court of Justice 1996) the ICJ could find neither any specific authorization in international law of the threat or use of nuclear weapons, nor a comprehensive prohibition of their use, but emphasized that any possible use must be compatible

Table 7.1 Key multilateral arms control treaties

Treaty	Entry into force	Provisions
Partial test ban treaty	1963	Bans nuclear tests except underground
Non-proliferation treaty	1970	For non-nuclear-weapon states: receive civil nuclear technology in return for not acquiring nuclear weapons For nuclear-weapon-states: pledge to nuclear disarmament by negotiation
Biological and toxin weapons convention	1975	Bans development, stockpiling or use of biological weapons: convention currently no provision for verification
Convention on certain conventional weapons (Inhumane weapons convention)	1980	Bans exploding weapons that leave x-ray lucent fragments; certain types of landmines; incendiary weapons designed to set fire to targets; blinding lasers
UN convention on the rights of the child	1989	Parties: respect humanitarian law in armed conflict relevant to the child; ensure that persons under fifteen years do not take part in hostilities and are not recruited into armed forces; promote physical and psychological recovery of child victims of armed conflict
Chemical weapons convention	1997	Bans development, stockpiling or use of chemical weapons; sets up Organization for Prevention of Chemical Warfare
Landmines convention	1998	Forbids production, distribution, stockpiling or use of anti-personnel mines; calls for destruction of existing stocks
Comprehensive test ban treaty	?	Banning all nuclear test explosions; awaiting key ratifications before entry into force

with existing international law, such as avoiding disproportionate harm to civilians and neutrals. The Court could not rule out use 'in an extreme circumstance of self-defence, in which the very survival of a State would be at stake'. It concluded that, under Article VI of the Non-Proliferation Treaty (Table 7.1) 'There exists an obligation. . .to bring to a conclusion negotiations leading to nuclear disarmament. . .under effective international control' – in other words, agreement on a nuclear weapons convention.

A nuclear weapons convention

Chemical and biological weapons are forbidden under existing international conventions (see below). IPPNW, with other NGOs and in collaboration with the govern-

Table 7.2 Selected medical war-related organizations

Organization	Activities and objectives	Address
International Committee of Red Cross	Medical and humanitarian relief in war zones, liaison with prisoners of war. Politically neutral	19 Ave de la Paix CH–1202 Geneva Switzerland
International Physicians for Prevention of Nuclear War	Prevention of nuclear war by elimination of nuclear weapons and other weapons of mass destruction; more recently prevention of all war. Umbrella group with affiliates in 60 countries	126 Rogers Street Cambridge MA 02142 USA
Médecins sans Frontières	Assisting populations in distress, particularly victims of armed conflicts. Neutral, aims to work with governments in power, but believes rights of populations in danger supersede national sovereignty and will undertake 'cross-border' operations	39 Rue de la Tourelle B-1040 Brussels Belgium
Physicians for Human Rights	Investigates and publicizes breaches of human rights in conflict zones, including inappropriate use of weapons (landmines), ethnic cleansing, torture	100 Boylston Street Boston MA 02116 USA

ments of sympathetic middle-ranking states (Green 1999), is concentrating its activities on achieving a similar convention for nuclear weapons, which would make the production, testing, stockpiling, or use of nuclear weapons illegal. This is feasible as well as desirable (Rotblat 1998); a draft convention has been drawn up (Datan and Ware 1999) and has been deposited as a United Nations (UN) document by Costa Rica. Meanwhile, until such a convention is achieved, the risk of accidental nuclear war can be reduced by an agreement among the nuclear powers not to be the first to use nuclear weapons and to take them off high alert. Attempts are in progress to achieve a treaty banning the production of weapons-usable fissile material. In the longer term, provided the world's energy needs can be supplied sustainably in other ways (Chapter 5), civil nuclear power, which produces plutonium, should be phased out and plutonium and other nuclear waste safely disposed of – a problem which currently has no obvious solution.

At the April–May 2000 review conference of the Non-Proliferation Treaty, the five nuclear-weapon-states parties gave an unconditional commitment to the global elimination of nuclear weapons. Shortly before this, Russia ratified the Comprehensive Test Ban Treaty (which the USA has signed but not ratified). However, President Putin has threatened to withdraw its ratification and its undertakings under the second Strategic Arms Reduction Treaty if the USA proceeds with the plans for ballistic missile defence to which President George W Bush is apparently strongly committed.

Chemical and biological warfare

With nuclear weapons, chemical and biological warfare (CBW) agents are classified, in view of their potentially widespread and indiscriminate effects, as weapons of mass destruction. Many regard them as 'the poor countries' nuclear weapons'.

Chemical weapons

Chemical weapons were first used in World War 1, causing some 50 000 deaths and over a million casualties. The horror they generated led to their being restricted by the 1925 Geneva protocol; this outlawed use but not stockpiling, and several states entered reservations to the protocol allowing use in retaliation. Japan used chemical weapons in China between 1938 and 1945. Both the allies and other Axis powers accumulated large stockpiles, but none were otherwise used in World War 2. Their use by Iraq against its Kurdish population caused several thousand deaths, and many deaths and thousands of casualties may have occurred in the first (Iran–Iraq) Gulf war.

Chemical agents fall into two groups, non-lethal and lethal. Non-lethal agents such as CS gas are used for riot control. Lethal agents include the nerve gases (sarin, soman, tabun, VX), which are non-competitive blockers of cholinesterase, can be absorbed both through lungs and skin, and cause death by respiratory paralysis. They are among the most potent poisons known, fatal in milligram amounts; sarin was used by the Japanese terrorist group Aum Shinrikyo in its attack on the Tokyo underground railway, with 12 deaths and hundreds of casualties. Chlorine, phosgene, and sulphur mustard are vesicants and cause severe pulmonary oedema; sulphur mustard damages deoxyribonucleic acid (DNA) and is a carcinogen (Maynard and Marrs 1996).

The Chemical Weapons Convention

The Chemical Weapons Convention (CWC), which took some 20 years to negotiate, was signed in 1993 and entered into force in 1997. It now has over 125 signatories, but several states suspected of having or wanting chemical warfare (CW) capability are not parties, including some in the middle east. The CWC provides for destruction of chemical weapons, CW protection facilities, and for the prevention of the re-emergence of CW through its verification system. Destruction of existing stocks will not be easy given the toxicity of the substances involved, and there are fears that the Russian Federation in particular may fall behind in its obligations. Operations under the CWC are monitored by the Organization for Prohibition of Chemical Weapons based at The Hague, which so far seems to be fulfilling its planned function (Developments in the Organization for the Prohibition of Chemical Weapons 1999); medically trained personnel are among its staff.

Biological warfare

Biological warfare (BW) is deliberately inducing disease. Bio-war antedates the germ theory of disease, and may, for instance, have led to the outbreak of the Black Death. Tartars besieging the port of Caffa in the Crimea in 1346 were attacked by plague, but before leaving catapulted some of their dead over the city walls. Some of the inhabitants fled to Genoa, but took the disease with them. In 1763, British soldiers deliberately passed smallpox-contaminated blankets to North American Indians. The Hague Peace Conferences of 1899 and 1905 condemned bio-warfare, but Germany used anthrax in World War 1, though primarily on livestock (British Medical Association 1999). Use, but not stockpiling, of biological weapons was forbidden under the 1925 Geneva Convention, but as with CW, several states entered reservations allowing retaliation.

Some research on BW was carried out in Germany in the 1930s, and anthrax was stockpiled by the UK in World War 2. Research, including gruesome experiments on Chinese prisoners, was more extensive in Japan (British Medical Association 1999). After World War 2 there was a major programme in the USA, and at least eight agents were weaponized (Hay 1999*a,b*). The programme was abandoned because of the realization that BW would be an effective force for poorer countries that could not afford nuclear weapons, so that an effective ban on BW was regarded as more important. The outcome, the Biological and Toxin Weapons Convention (BTWC) (Table 7.1) of 1972, bans both stockpiling and use of BW, but contains no provision for verification. Research and development continued nevertheless in several countries party to the BTWC. A serious programme continued in the Soviet Union, with weaponization of viral agents, and the use of genetic engineering (British Medical Association 1999). It is now clear that an outbreak of anthrax in Sverdlovsk originated in a BW facility. Since the second Gulf War, the extent of Iraq's BW programme has also come to light. Biological weapons could also be used by terrorist groups; Aum Shinrikyo experimented with a variety of pathogens.

Today's threats encompass the full range of biologically active agents: viruses (smallpox, Ebola virus); bacteria (anthrax, plague, tularaemia); bacterial and other toxins (aflatoxin, botulinum toxin, ricin) (British Medical Association 1999). The route of attack would be by inhalation; it has been claimed (Office of Technology Assessment 1993) that a single attack with anthrax on a major city could kill one to three million, more than a nuclear attack. Toxins, which are covered by both the CWC and the BTWC, could be used as either battlefield weapons or as a terror weapon against population centres. Misuse of modern biotechnology is a worrying possibility; genes for pathogenicity from, say, plague bacteria could be genetically engineered into non-pathogenic organisms such as *Escherichia coli*, or genes for antibiotic resistance into standard pathogens (British Medical Association 1999). Attacking crops with biological agents is a realistic possibility, and could cause mass starvation in areas highly dependent upon single food crops such as rice (Rogers *et al.* 1999).

As already noted, the 1972 BTWC contains no provision for verification. The convention is due for review in 2001, and work has been in progress for several years on an additional protocol to make good this lack. There are hopes that agreement on a text can be achieved in 2001 (Pearson 2000). A principal difficulty is the need for regular inspections of biotechnology facilities. These can be used either for legitimate microbiological research (permitted of course under the BWTC), some with important commercial implications, or for work on BW agents. As much biotechnology research is in the USA, the attitude of its government (and its response to pressure from the biotechnology industry) is critical to the achievement of a verification protocol. The co-operation of the chemical industry in verification of the CWC has set an encouraging precedent.

The ethics of work on biotechnology is a matter for individuals as well as corporations. Speaking with respect to nuclear weapons, Professor Sir Joseph Rotblat, in his Nobel Prize acceptance speech (Rotblat 1999), called for the equivalent of the Hippocratic oath for scientists to include refusal to work on nuclear weapons, and recognition of the importance of whistle blowing as a human right of scientists. Few doctors now take the Hippocratic oath on qualifying, but the opportunity should be available for all health workers to refuse to work on the application of biotechnology to bio-war (though work on vaccination against possible pathogens would have to be an exception). Similarly, the opportunity to formally reject participation in CW research (for pharmacologists) and on newer conventional weapons (pathologists and others – see below) should be available.

Influential organizations, both nationally (such as the British Medical Association) and internationally (the WHO) should also work towards the elimination of weapons of mass destruction by bringing pressure on their own governments and calling for stronger international agreements. Vigilance will be needed for a long time, the development of nuclear physics led to nuclear weapons, and progress in chemistry to chemical weapons, while developments in biotechnology leading to bacterial pathogens targeted against specific ethnic groups are a sinister possibility for the future (British Medical Association 1999). Advances in science and technology, as yet only the stuff of science fiction, will have possibilities for harm as well as good.

Conventional weapons

Apart from the casualties from chemical warfare in the first Gulf war, all the 20 million or more war-related deaths since the end of World War 2 have been due to 'conventional' weapons. These range from fuel–air missiles, with a destructive power of the same order as low-yield nuclear weapons, through warplanes, battle tanks, artillery and land mines, to small arms. The wars in which conventional weapons are used may involve major powers, as in Vietnam, Afghanistan, former Yugoslavia, and Chechnya, but are more often intrastate conflicts, between a government and rebels, or between factions within a state. The number of conflicts actually increased after the end of the cold war, with over 50 in 1992, then falling to just over 30 per year, but perhaps increasing again (Wallensteen and Sollenberg 1999).

'Superfluous Injury or Unnecessary Suffering'

The concept that the damaging effect of a weapon system should not be excessive dates back to the 1899 Hague Peace Conference. It is distinct from the clear prohibition under international law of indiscriminate attacks on civilians, and refers to the extent of injury to survivors caused by the weapon (length of stay in hospital, number of transfusions or amputations, extent of permanent disability, etc.).

The International Committee of the Red Cross (ICRC) has accumulated a large database on war wounded treated in its field hospitals (Coupland 1996; Coupland and Korver 1991). The ICRC's 'Superfluous Injury or Unnecessary Suffering' (SIrUS)

Project seeks to prohibit under international humanitarian law any weapon system with excessive effects by these criteria (Coupland 1997). Weapons which could be outlawed might include cluster bombs, napalm, and fuel–air weapons. Laser weapons deliberately designed to cause blindness (Doswald Beck 1993) have been banned under the Convention on Certain Conventional Weapons (the Inhumane Weapons Convention, Table 7.1) though not laser range-finders that happen to blind as a 'side effect'. The case of land mines is described in Box 7.1.

Box 7.1: **Anti-personnel land mines: a case study in presentation**

The successful outcome of the campaign to ban anti-personnel mines shows the value of well-informed co-operation between medical and other NGOs and sympathetic governments. The campaign can be divided into four phases, the last still in progress.

Awareness

Reports from medical groups (Coupland and Korver 1991; Human Rights Watch Arms Project and Physicians for Human Rights 1993) described the effects of land mines, in particular the high rate of death and disability, wound complications, and proportion of children and other civilians injured.

Publicity

Collaboration with other NGOs, especially Oxfam, and skilled presentation in the media, generated widespread public concern. Active support from well-known public figures, particularly Princess Diana, contributed greatly.

Obtaining a treaty . . .

Use of some types of anti-personnel mines was limited under the Inhumane Weapons Convention. Continued public pressure, and increasing support from sympathetic governments, led to the signature of the 1997 Ottawa Convention prohibiting the use, stockpiling, production, and transfer of all types, with provision for their destruction.

. . . and after

To be of maximal value, a treaty must be universal; China, Russia and the USA have not signed the Ottawa Convention. De-mining, and physical and psychosocial rehabilitation of victims will be needed for many years.

Information: International Campaign to Ban Landmines Resource Centre, Osterhausgt 27, N–0183 Oslo, Norway

The approach of the SIrUS Project has, predictably, been criticized from both sides. Although they have to 'pick up the pieces', many military doctors still support the ability of their active service colleagues to be as 'effective' as possible, while anti-militarists are concerned that specifically outlawing certain weapons automatically legitimizes others. At the very least, though, health professionals working on weapons effects should carefully consider their ethical position if their efforts promote the development and use of weapons infringing the SIrUS criteria.

War in the twenty-first century: new challenges to health?

The second Gulf war and wars in former Yugoslavia warn of new health hazards from armed intervention by forces of the most developed countries. To minimize casualties to themselves, these forces use high-level precision bombing and missiles – not all accurately, resulting in bomb victims reminiscent of World War 2. Both the targets hit, and the bombs and missiles used, disseminate various toxic substances harming both combatants and non-combatants. In the Gulf, there were few direct combat casualties, but a large number of allied military have since become ill for currently unexplained reasons. In Iraq, the aftermath of damage to power, sanitation, and water supplies, together with economic sanctions, have devastated health care, and cancers and birth defects may have increased. Some of the factors blamed for these 'Gulf War illnesses' are listed in Table 7.3. In former Yugoslavia, targeting of oil refineries liberated large amounts of toxic chemicals. Targeting power facilities imperils hospitals, especially intensive care units. In the future, 'cyber-warfare' on modern computer networks could also paralyse hospitals, as well as the military.

Table 7.3 Possible causative factors in Gulf war illnesses

Factor	Comment
In allied veterans: Vaccines	Multiple, rapidly given, against tropical diseases and BW agents
Toxic smoke	Burning oil wells
Insecticides	Organophosphates; sprayed inside tents
CW agents	May have been liberated by bombing of Iraqi munition dumps
Protectives against CW	e.g. pyridostigmine
Depleted uranium In Iraqis:	See text
Lack of health care	Destruction of infrastructure; sanctions
Depleted uranium	See text
CW agents	Late effect of use in first Gulf war (mustard gas is a carcinogen and mutagen)

It is unlikely, despite the chemical toxicity and radioactivity of depleted uranium, that its use in large amounts in the Gulf war, or more recently in the Balkans, is responsible for the effects claimed by some (Fetter and von Hippel 1999). Nevertheless, the indiscriminate use of missiles containing a toxic and radioactive substance should be banned under the Inhumane Weapons Convention.

'Non-lethal' weapons

Modern technology is being applied to a variety of weapons designed as incapacitating rather than lethal. These include lasers and other optical 'munitions', acoustic weapons, electromagnetic pulse transmitters ('cyber-weapons'), and non-lethal agents, chemicals, and immobilizers such as foams and nets (Lewer and Schofield 1997). There are medical objections to the use of many of these; blinding lasers are, as noted, banned under the Inhumane Weapons Convention. Some are far from non-lethal, either directly (acoustic weapons (Arkin 1997)) or indirectly (cyber-warfare, see above). 'Non-lethal' agents, including chemicals such as CS gas and immobilizers, are widely used by paramilitaries for riot control. As such, they are of particular attraction to governments with dubious human rights records. A loophole in the CWC could be interpreted as permitting the development of 'calmative' or 'sleep' agents acting directly on the nervous system. The market for these agents is obvious, but should clearly be very strictly limited by codes of conduct for the arms trade (see below).

Small arms

Wars between developing countries and intrastate conflicts, like most of the wars of the second half of the twentieth century, will continue to be fought largely with small arms. There are two aspects to the problem, conflicts of interest between individual countries, particularly in the developing world, and opposition within them, but also the free availability of weapons to settle the differences violently. It has been suggested that there are 500 million firearms in circulation worldwide (Renner 1997), over 100 million of them semi-automatic rifles such as the AK 47 or Kalashnikov, which in some parts of Africa can be purchased for the price of a chicken or a goat. Around 200 million firearms are owned privately in the USA. In Africa in particular, when one conflict goes into remission, many of the arms used are sold on the black market to participants in the next (Renner 1997). Arms used in these conflicts also include machine guns, sub-machine guns, mortars, and anti-tank weapons.

Civilian casualties

A feature of the casualties from these conflicts is the high proportion of non-combatants, including women and children. Figures of 80 per cent or more civilian casualties may be too high (Meddings 2001), but this does not make lower figures acceptable. Many civilian deaths and injuries from small arms occur well after the end of active conflict, from 'casual' or accidental use of firearms left in the houses of former combatants (including by children). Others result from detonation of left-over munitions, including shells and cluster bombs but particularly land mines. Large tracts of otherwise cultivable land in some least-developed countries are unusable until cleared of land mines, and at times of food shortage the temptation to take a chance with using these areas can be irresistible. Loss of livestock contributes to food shortages.

In least-developed countries, disruption of health care from poverty resulting from war (and deliberate destruction of what facilities exist) is a major but unquantifiable 'side effect' of conflict.

Disposing of small arms

Essential as it is, curbs on the official arms trade from industrialized to developing world are not enough, and there have been a variety of approaches to the disposal of weapons. Medical relief and rehabilitation organizations working in combat zones, with other NGOs, can participate in the newly formed International Action Network on Small Arms (Table 7.4), both to curb the arms trade and to promote local initiatives to collect and destroy weapons from war zones before they are recycled. Attempts to link arms disposal with UN peace-keeping operations have been a failure (Renner 1997); local 'buy-back' schemes, in which arms are bought at just above the 'black market' rate, perhaps in kind rather than for cash, have been more successful. Such schemes can be linked to programmes for reintegrating the many thousands of ex-soldiers back into society (Renner 1997), and to the provision or restoration of health care facilities.

Children and war

Children are both direct and indirect victims of war (Machel 1996). They are killed and injured, with other non-combatants, by straying into the line of fire or into minefields, and are psychologically traumatized by growing up in war zones. Many

Table 7.4 International NGO collaboration for disarmament

Coalition	Objective	Address
Global Action to Prevent War	A four-phase process for successive treaties to increase transparency on armed forces and military spending; substantial cuts in armed forces; a permanent transfer to the UN of authority and capability for intervention to prevent or end war	c/o Institute for Defence & Disarmament Studies 675 Massachusetts Ave Cambridge MA 02139 USA
International Action Network on Small Arms	Raising awareness of the impact of small arms; campaigning for an international code of conduct on arms exports; reintegrating former combatants into society	Box 422 37 Store Street London WC1E 7BS UK
Coalition to Stop the Use of Child Soldiers	Stopping the use of children in armed conflict; rehabilitating former child soldiers; raising recruitment age to 18	11–13 Chemin des Anenomes CH 1219 Geneva Switzerland

are orphaned, separated from their families, or become refugees (Chapter 9). Some, for sheer survival, end up in military camps, where the girls often become sex objects and the boys child soldiers, sometimes under ten years of age. Modern semi-automatic rifles are very light and easy to handle, and are manageable by children of this age. Other children, in Africa in particular, are abducted by armed militias and brutally inducted into their ranks, or mutilated if reluctant. Physical and psychological rehabilitation of child soldiers will be a major task for health services for many years.

Indirectly, children suffer disproportionately from malnutrition and diarrhoeal diseases around war zones. Immunization programmes are difficult or impossible to organize in conflict-torn areas – the Horn of Africa is the last refuge of poliomyelitis.

All this means that most countries at war are overtly breaching the UN Convention on the Rights of the Child (Table 7.1). Under this convention, the minimum age for military service is 15. At its 2000 General Assembly, the UN approved an Optional Protocol, promoted by UNICEF and others, raising the minimum age to 18 (Table 7.4). The UK, which recruits at 16, has ratified this protocol, but its policy will be unchanged, on the grounds that recruitment of 16–17-year-olds is voluntary and with parental consent. The government is no doubt well aware that eighteen-year-olds are sufficiently more mature to make recruitment more difficult – which would force a revision of what activities the military can undertake.

The arms industry and the arms trade

At the height of the cold war world arms spending reached US$1 trillion annually. It has fallen to about US$700 billion, but the rate of fall may be slowing down (Bonn International Center for Conversion 1998). This represents some 3 per cent of global gross domestic product. The UK currently spends about UK£22 billion annually, which supports 1.5 million jobs, including suppliers and sub-contractors as well as military personnel. Official arms transfers also peaked during the cold war, but fell from about US$60 billion in 1987 to between US$18 and 23 billion in the mid–1990s (Bonn International Center for Conversion 1998; Sivard 1996), largely due to the collapse of the economy of the former Soviet Union. (Figures for ex-USSR arms sales are based on Central Intelligence Agency estimates of previous exports, which may be exaggerated, so that the fall may have been overestimated.) The five permanent members of the UN Security Council (USA, Russia, UK, France, and China) are responsible for over 80 per cent of official arms exports. The extent of unofficial transfers of small arms is unknown and probably unknowable.

Even if it is not used for actual fighting, military spending is economically and environmentally harmful, and the money is not available for purposes such as education and health care (Sidel 1995). Developed countries are having difficulty coping with increasing demands for health care, while many developing countries are unable to provide even basic care for much of their population. For instance, the programme of the 1994 Cairo Conference on Reproductive Health and Development was costed at US$17 billion annually – just over one week's world arms spending.

Protagonists of high military spending and the arms trade justify them by reference to the right of national self-defence under Article 51 of the UN Charter – but forget that self-defence is only intended as a temporary measure before referring disputes to the Security Council. Some also justify arms trading on the basis that 'if we didn't do it, someone else would' – scarcely the high moral ground.

Alternatives

There have been many different approaches to achieving a peaceful world, falling into three main groups (Rapoport 1999). The pacifist sees the origins of war in the human psyche, while peace making (conflict resolution) attempts to resolve specific disputes between states or factions. The central goal for the abolitionist is war as an institution. The medical response involves elements of all three.

The public and decision makers must be informed of the effects of war, as in the land mines campaign (Box 7.1) or by IPPNW for nuclear weapons. Mikhail Gorbachev was influenced by IPPNW to begin his efforts to reverse the nuclear arms race (Gorbachev 1987). Medical bodies should collaborate with other NGOs and sympathetic governments and national medical groups can work through the WHO.

Disarmament

Medical bodies can support various projects towards disarmament (Table 7.4). For instance, Global Action to Prevent War, of which IPPNW is a sponsor, presents a radical but practicable programme for a four-phase reduction of conventional armaments over several years, with progressive transfer of control over powers of military intervention to the UN. For health professionals, achievement of a major degree of disarmament would free huge human, financial, and material resources for the provision of better health care.

A priority is cutting the supply of arms to trouble zones. The European Union (EU) has established a code of conduct to do this; the UN has only a register of major arms transfers (planes, tanks, artillery, etc.), that could be widened to incorporate many more categories of arms and a worldwide code of conduct. In view of its large share of the world economy, conversion of the arms industry to peaceful purposes is a key part of this process. Many schemes are now in operation (Bonn International Center for Conversion 1998), and are achieving a measure of success (Brzoska 1999). As noted already, disposal of the huge number of light weapons already in circulation, and recycled from conflict to conflict by the black market, may be best achieved at local level (Renner 1997).

Common security

The replacement for war as an institution already exists; it is called the UN. In a changing world, and already expanded from 51 states to over 180, some reforms are needed to enable the UN, as the preamble of its charter states, 'to save future generations from the scourge of war'. Space does not permit detailed discussion of this subject, and medical groups go beyond their expertise in pressing for reform, but one point at least is clear. The WHO, which is part of the UN system and is already contributing directly to peace building (Lancet 2000) must include in its remit both the needs of the global health system, and the demonstration that war and the proportion of the world's resources diverted to preparations for war prevent these needs being fulfilled.

Permanent membership of the UN Security Council should be expanded to include more representatives from the developing world. The veto powers of the permanent members of the Security Council should be modified so that the council can function more effectively (Carnegie Commission on Preventing Deadly Conflict 1992; Commission on Global Governance 1995). The role of the International Court of Justice should also be extended; all member states of the UN should be obliged to accept its jurisdiction in the peaceful settlement of disputes – not, as now, only when it suits them. The court has settled many disagreements, which in the past could have led to war and all interstate disputes that could lead to war should be automatically referred to it (Higgins 2000). National governments in their policies should be encouraged towards common security rather than their own short-term interests, as the US is currently doing with its plans for ballistic missile defence which threaten to halt progress towards nuclear disarmament. The WHO should regularly ask the Court for advisory opinions on the legality of international actions and activities that have a significant impact on health and the provision of health care.

Intrastate wars – the majority, as already noted – present difficulties for the UN. On the one hand, Article 2.7 of its Charter forbids it to intervene in matters 'within the domestic jurisdiction of any state.' On the other, the Security Council is permitted to intervene if it considers that internal conflicts present a threat to international security. The extent to which national sovereignty is sacrosanct needs clarification (Carnegie Commission on Preventing Deadly Conflict 1992; Commission on Global Governance 1995) but intervention breaching it should be restricted to a reformed Security Council.

The manner of intervention is also problematic. As in Iraq and former Yugoslavia, resort to war leaves behind as many problems as it solves, but the use of extensive economic sanctions is also unsatisfactory, causing serious adverse effects on health (Gottstein 1999). There must be much more frequent and early resort to preventive diplomacy by the UN, preferably mediated through its regional bodies such as the Organization of African Unity or the Organization for Security and Co-operation in Europe. Concerns of health workers at a local level could reach these more easily than the UN itself. The UN's spending on preventive diplomacy is tiny, and diversion of quite a small proportion of arms spending in its direction would save much suffering.

There has been a huge increase in international law, in the UN system and in the European Union, concerned with the issues raised in other chapters of this book. Arms control and disarmament law should be similarly promoted. Legal constraints must restrict the range of potential disputes that could degenerate into conflict – 'law not war'.

The causes of war

The ultimate in prevention must be dealing with the underlying causes of war such as environmental threats, poverty, and resource depletion. Further conflicts could develop over water, which is vital for health and sanitation. Debt relief, as well as being positively linked to provision of education and health care, should be conditional on cuts by the beneficiary in military spending. In the fourth century AD, the Roman Vegetius wrote '*qui desiderat pacem, praeparet bellum*' (if you want peace, prepare for war'). As he wrote, the empire was in decline, in large part from supporting a huge standing army in constant border wars. Today's slogan should be 'if you want peace, prepare for peace'. A detailed programme was presented at the May 1999 Hague Appeal for Peace, again a joint initiative involving IPPNW (UN 1999). Health workers have a key role in implementing such initiatives – and making the world a healthier place at the same time. (MacQueen *et al.* 2001)

Acknowledgements

I am very grateful to Sandra Watt of the Education Centre Library, Ashford Hospital, Middlesex for obtaining source material, and to Professor Malcolm Dando and Drs Frank Barnaby, Alastair Hay, and Liz Waterston for helpful comments on earlier drafts.

References

Arkin, W. M. (1997) Acoustic antipersonnel weapons: an inhumane future? *Medicine, Conflict and Survival,* **13,** 314–26.

Bonn International Center for Conversion (1998) *Conversion survey 1998.* Oxford University Press, Oxford.

British Medical Association (1999) *Biotechnology, weapons and humanity.* Harwood, Amsterdam.

British Medical Association Board of Science and Education (1983) *The medical effects of nuclear war.* John Wiley, Chichester.

Brzoska, M. (1999) Military conversion: the balance sheet. *Journal of Peace Research,* **36,** 131–40.

Carnegie Commission on Preventing Deadly Conflict (1992) Preventing deadly conflict. Final report. Carnegie Commission, Washington DC.

Commission on Global Governance (1995) *Our global neighbourhood.* Oxford University Press. Oxford.

Coupland, R. M. (1996) The effect of weapons: defining superfluous injury and unnecessary suffering. *Medicine and Global Survival,* **3,** A1.

Coupland, R. M. (1997) *The SIrUS Project.* International Committee of the Red Cross, Geneva.

Coupland, R. M. and Korver, A. (1991) Injuries from antipersonnel mines: the experience of the International Committee of the Red Cross. *British Medical Journal,* **303,** 1509–12.

Datan, M. and Ware, A. (1999) *Security and survival: the case for a nuclear weapons convention.* IPPNW/IALANA//.INESAP, Cambridge, MA.

Developments in the Organization for the Prohibition of Chemical Weapons (1999) *CBW Conventions Bulletin,* **43,** March 2–10. SPRU, University of Sussex, Sussex.

Doswald Beck, L. (1993) *Blinding weapons.* International Committee of the Red Cross, Geneva.

Fetter, S. and Hippel F. von (1999) When the dust settles. *Bulletin of The Atomic Scientists,* **55**(6), 42–45.

Forrow, L., Blair, B. G., Helfand, I. *et al.* (1998) Accidental nuclear war – a post-car war assessment. *New England Journal of Medicine,* **338**, 1326–31.

Gorbachev, M. (1987) *Perestroika.* Collins, London.

Gottstein, U. (1999) Peace through sanctions? Lessons from Cuba, former Yugoslavia and Iraq, *Medicine Conflict and Survival,* **15**, 271–85.

Green, R. D. (1999) *Fast track to zero nuclear weapons: the Middle Powers Initiative.* MPI, Cambridge, MA.

Groebel, J. and Hinde, R. A. (1989) *Aggression and war: their biological and social bases.* Cambridge University Press, Cambridge.

Harwell, M. A. and Hutchinson, T. C. (1985) *Environmental consequences of nuclear war, Vol. II, Ecological and agricultural effects.* John Wiley, Chichester.

Hay, A. (1999*a*) Simulants, stimulants and diseases: the evolution of the United States biological warfare programs, 1945–60. *Medicine, Conflict and Survival,* **15**, 198–214.

Hay, A. (1999*b*) A magic sword or a big itch: an historical look at the United States biological weapons programme. *Medicine, Conflict and Survival,* **15**, 215–34.

Higgins, R. (2000) 'To save succeeding generations from the scourge of war': the role of the International Court of Justice, *Medicine, Conflict and Survival,* **16**, 61–72.

Hinde, R. A. and Watson, H. E. (1995) *War – a cruel necessity? The basis of institutionalised violence.* IB Tauris, London.

Human Rights Watch Arms Project and Physicians for Human Rights (1993) *Landmines: a deadly legacy.* Human Rights Watch, New York.

International Court of Justice (1996) Advisory opinion: legality of the threat or use of nuclear weapons. Doc A/51/218. UN, New York.

Lancet (2000) Defining the limits of public health. *The Lancet,* **355**, 587.

Lewer, N. (1992) *Physicians and the peace movement.* Frank Cass, London.

Lewer, N. and Schofield, S. (1997) *Non-lethal weapons: a fatal attraction?* Zed Books, London.

Machel, G. (1996) Impact of armed conflict on children. Report submitted pursuant to GA resolution 48/157. UN, New York.

Mac Queen G., Santa-Barbara J., Neufeld V. *et al.* (2001) Health and peace: time for a new discipline. *Lancet,* **357**, 1460–61.

Maynard, R. L. and Marrs, T. C. (1996) Poisoning in conflict. In *Oxford textbook of medicine,* 3rd edn, ed. D. J. Weatherall, J. G. C. Ledingham, and D. A. Warrell. Oxford University Press, Oxford.

Meddings D. R. (2001) Civilians and war. *Medicine, Conflict and Survival,* **17**, 6–16.

Office of Technology Assessment (1993) Proliferation of weapons of mass destruction: Assessing the risk. OTA-ISC–559. United States Congress, Washington DC.

Pearson, G. S. (2000) Preventing deliberate disease. *Medicine, Conflict and Survival,* **16**, 43–60.

Physicians for Social Responsibility (1962) The medical consequences of thermonuclear war. *New England Journal of Medicine,* **266**, 1126–55.

Pittock, A. B., Ackerman, T. P., Crutzen, P. J. *et al* (1985) *Environmental consequences of nuclear war,* Vol. 1, *physical and atmospheric effects.* John Wiley, Chichester.

Rapoport, A. (1999) From a nuclear-free to a war-free world. In *Ending war: the force of reason,* ed. M. Bruce and T. Milne. Macmillan, Basingstoke.

Renner, M. (1997) *Small arms, big impact: the next challenge of disarmament.* Worldwatch Institute, Washington DC.

Rogers, P., Whitby, S., and Dando, M. (1999) Biological warfare against crops. *Scientific American,* **280**(6), 62–7.

Rotblat, J. (1998) *Nuclear weapons: the road to zero.* Westview, Oxford.

Rotblat, J. (1999) Remember your humanity. In *Ending war: the force of reason,* ed. M. Bruce and T. Milne. Macmillan, Basingstoke.

Sidel, V. W. (1995) The international arms trade and its impact on health. *British Medical Journal,* **311,** 1677–80.

Sidel, V. W. and Levy, D. (1997) *War and public health.* Oxford University Press, Oxford.

Sivard, R. L. (1991) *World military and social expenditures 1991.* World Priorities, Washington DC.

Sivard, R. L. (1996) *World military and social expenditures 1996.* World Priorities, Washington DC.

UN (1999) The Hague agenda for peace and justice for the 21st century. UN Document A/54/98. UN, New York.

Wallensteen, P. and Sollenberg, M. (1999) Armed conflict, 1989–98. *Journal of Peace Research,* **36,** 593–606.

WHO Management Group (1983, 1987) *Effects of nuclear war on health and health services.* 1st and 2nd edn. WHO, Geneva.

Wright, E. G. (2000) Inducible genomic instability: new insights into the biological effects of ionising radiation. *Medicine, Conflict and Survival,* **16,** 119–32.

Chapter 8

Confronting the tobacco epidemic: emerging mechanisms of global governance

Heather Wipfli, Douglas W. Bettcher, Chitra Subramaniam, and Allyn L. Taylor

Introduction

The worldwide struggle against tobacco illustrates how existing mechanisms of governance can be used in new and innovative ways to address a global threat to health. At the 52nd World Health Assembly in May 1999, the 191 Member States of the World Health Organization (WHO) adopted, by consensus, a resolution that started a process leading toward formal negotiations on a WHO Framework Convention on Tobacco Control (FCTC) – a new treaty designed to circumscribe the global rise and spread of the tobacco epidemic. Formal negotiations on the convention began in October 2000. The adoption of the convention and key protocols is targeted for completion by the year 2003. This historic resolution marks the first time the member states of the WHO have harnessed the organization's capacity to develop binding international conventions or agreements to protect and promote global public health.

The FCTC offers a unique opportunity for the public health community to institutionalize their influence and views through the negotiation of a binding treaty text. Once adopted and entered into force, the FCTC may serve as an effective instrument for counteracting the globalization of the tobacco epidemic by serving as a platform for multi-lateral commitment, co-operation, and action to address the rise and spread of tobacco consumption. However, the significance of the FCTC lies not only in the treaty itself, but in 'the power of the process' (Taylor 2000).

The treaty-making process has extended the tobacco control dialogue to numerous governing structures which had not been accessed by the public health community before. Within governments, the development of the FCTC has created the opportunity for tobacco control to expand to ministries other than health, including foreign affairs, trade, and agriculture. Multi-sectoral co-operation, both on the national and global level, is enhancing partnerships and broadening the scientific evidence base in support of a global regulatory framework for tobacco. In addition, public support for tobacco control has been enhanced through activities such as the first ever WHO public hearings, aggressive advocacy campaigns and international conferences. These activities stimulate public opinion and national action, which may result in dramatic contributions to curtailing the spiralling pandemic before the consensus on global tobacco norms is secured (Taylor 2000).

This chapter traces the development of the FCTC and its impact on the development of global tobacco governance. The chapter accomplishes four tasks. First, it examines the main trends in the international tobacco environment that demand co-ordinated global action to combat the growing epidemic. Second, it examines how the concept of global governance offers a framework in which health concerns, such as tobacco, can be addressed and third it explores the various governing mechanisms being used throughout the FCTC process. Fourth, it concludes by exploring the broader role negotiating processes can play in strengthening global health governance and improving health worldwide, and stresses the importance of involving health professionals and the public health community in advancing a global public health movement for tobacco control.

By focusing on the mechanisms of global governance, this chapter aims to provide public health professionals with new ways to complement local and international tobacco control initiatives. Moreover, the FCTC process outlined in this chapter provides an example of how various governing structures can be used to expand the reach of public health professionals in promoting various health issues. The FCTC process not only represents a ground-breaking moment in global tobacco control, but also represents a pathfinder for international co-operation in the twenty-first century.

Globalization of the tobacco epidemic

Current situation

Serious medical and scientific attention on the health consequences of smoking began in the 1950s (Doll and Hill 1954). This was largely a reflection of the development of epidemiology and the relatively modest number of victims claimed by tobacco prior to the twentieth century (Chaloupka and Warner 1998). Prior to the mid-twentieth century, relatively few people reached the ages at which tobacco takes its greatest toll (average life expectancy in the USA was 47 in 1900, in 1998 it was 75) (Chaloupka and Warner 1998). In addition, mass production and widespread use of the most dangerous form of tobacco consumption, cigarette smoking, began only in the very late 1800s.

Since the 1950s over 70 000 scientific articles have implicated smoking in a wide variety of ailments, constituting the largest and best documented literature linking any behaviour to disease in humans (US Department of Health Services 1994). Smoking is the cause of 25 major categories of fatal and disabling disease, including lung and other cancers, ischaemic heart disease and chronic respiratory diseases (US Department of Health and Human Services 1989). Epidemiological studies also indicate that maternal smoking increases chances for reduced birth weight, miscarriage, placenta previa, and pre-natal mortality (US Department of Health and Human Services 1990). Half of all long-term smokers will eventually be killed by tobacco, and of these, half will die during the productive years of middle age, losing 20 to 25 years of life (Peto *et al.* 1994).

Environmental tobacco smoke also causes disease in many exposed persons who do not consume tobacco products (US Environmental Protection Agency 1992). In children, environmental tobacco smoke has been causally associated with adverse effects on respiratory health including increased risk of more severe lower respiratory infections, middle ear disease, chronic respiratory symptoms, asthma, and a reduction in the rate of lung growth during childhood (WHO 1999a). In adults, environmental tobacco smoke exposure has been found to be the leading cause of lung cancer and a major cause of heart disease in non-smokers (US Environmental Protection Agency 1992).

All told, tobacco-related diseases are the single most important cause of preventable death in the world. In 1999, there were over 1.25 billion smokers in the world, representing one-third of the world's population aged 15 years and over (Corrao *et al.* 2000). Cigarette smoking and other forms of tobacco consumption kill four million people per year, or one person every eight seconds (WHO 1999b). Recent trends in tobacco consumption indicate rising prevalence rates among children, adolescents, and women and an earlier age of initiation. Based on these current trends, tobacco is expected to kill 8.4 million people per year by 2020, 70 per cent of these deaths occurring in developing countries (Peto *et al.* 1998).

The distribution of the burden of disease caused by tobacco is increasingly shifting from industrialized to transitional and developing countries. While the percentage of all deaths attributable to tobacco is forecast to remain constant for the next twenty years in established market economies, developing countries and transitional economics are expected to see significant increases in tobacco-related deaths. In China alone, annual smoking deaths are expected to rise from 1 million to 3 million in 2050 (Murray and Lopez 1996).

The worldwide tobacco epidemic is being spread and reinforced through a complex mix of rapidly changing factors, including trade liberalization, global marketing and communications, and foreign direct investment. The globalization of the transnational tobacco industry, and in particular its new focus on transitional and developing countries, is a significant contributor to the increased risk of tobacco-related diseases worldwide. Already in the 1960s, major trans-national tobacco companies targeted growing markets in Latin America. In the 1980s, the transnational tobacco companies extended their reach into the newly industrialized economies of Asia (Japan, South Korea, Taiwan, and Thailand). In the 1990s, tobacco production and consumption reached new heights as tobacco companies moved into eastern Europe, China, and Africa and increasingly targeted young persons and women (Connoly 1992).

Trade liberalization

The global reach of the trans-national tobacco industry has been enhanced by the recent wave of international trade liberalization, particularly the Uruguay Round of trade negotiations, which included for the first time, the liberalization of unmanufactured tobacco (Chaloupka and Corbett 1998). The Uruguay Round, concluded in 1994, established the World Trade Organization (WTO) and brought about an over-

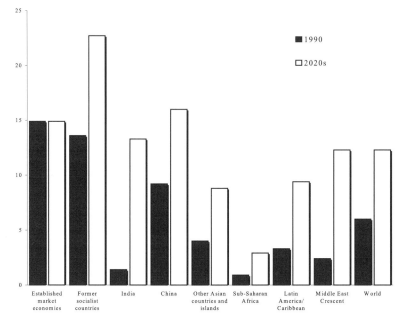

Figure 8.1 Percentage of all deaths attributable to tobacco

haul of the international trade regime by the conclusion of a number of new multi-lateral Agreements addressing contemporary trade issues, including tobacco. The new multi-lateral agreements of the WTO have facilitated the expansion of trade in tobacco products through significant reductions in tariff and non-tariff barriers to trade. Regional trade agreements and associations, such as the North American Free Trade Agreement, the European Union (EU), the Association of South-East Asian Nations, and the Common Market of Western African States, have acted in synergy with the global level by mandating further trade liberalization in goods and services including tobacco, at the regional level (Taylor and Bettcher 2000). Further, bilateral trade agreements, such as those negotiated in the 1980s by the US trade representative under Section 301 of the revised 1974 US Trade Act with Japan, Taiwan, and South Korea, have also facilitated market penetration in developing countries (Roemer 1993). The experience of Thailand in defending itself against tobacco company penetration is described in Box 8.1.

Trade liberalization has been linked to a greater risk of increased tobacco consumption, particularly in low- and middle-income countries. A recent study has empirically examined the relationship between cigarette consumption and global trade in tobacco products (Taylor *et al.* 2000). Conclusions from this study indicate that reduced trade barriers have had a large and significant impact on cigarette consumption in low-income countries, a small but significant impact in middle-income countries, and no significant impact in high income countries. The expected consequences of China's entry into the WTO are described in Box 8.2.

Box 8.1: **GATT 301 Thai cigarette case**

In April 1989, the trans-national tobacco companies called upon the US trade representative to Thailand to impose trade sanctions under Section 301, if Thailand continued to disallow market access to American cigarettes. The trans-national tobacco companies accused Thailand of using unfair trade practices against them, and demanded a completely free open market; freedom to establish their own market and distribution system; abolition of the high tax regime and discriminatory taxation; complete freedom to advertise and promote cigarettes through the press, radio, and television; and the right to sponsor sports and other events.

In December 1990, with the outcome of the bilateral talks between Thailand and the USA still inconclusive, the USA took the dispute to the General Agreement on Tariffs and Trade (GATT). The USA petitioned that Thailand's import ban and excise tax system were inconsistent with GATT rules. The American position was that the dispute was a national treatment issue, not a health issue and, therefore, Thailand should be ordered to remove unfair and discriminatory trade barriers that made it difficult for American products to compete with domestic products. Thailand's position was based on the health consequences of the market opening for cigarettes. Notably, health professionals were present on the Thai delegation. The Thai delegation persuaded the GATT panel to consult the WHO. The WHO team supported Thailand, arguing that foreign cigarette imports would have severe adverse health consequences.

In early September 1990, the GATT panel ruled that although Thailand's taxes on cigarettes were consistent with GATT, the import ban was nevertheless illegal. However, the ban on cigarette advertising was legal and Thailand could impose strict non-discriminatory labelling and ingredient disclosure regulations on cigarettes. In response, Thailand passed two very strong national tobacco control laws. The first, the Non-smokers' Health Promotion Act, outlawed smoking in public places and work places. The second, the Tobacco Products Control Act, included a complete ban on tobacco product advertising, on the sale of tobacco products to persons under 18 years old, on vending machines, and on the advertising of same name products, and outlawed many methods of promotion including exchanges and free sampling. Thailand is now one of only two countries in the world which require tobacco producers to disclose all ingredients in cigarettes on the package.

Source: Vaughan *et al.* 2000

In addition to trade liberalization, the trans-national tobacco companies have also taken advantage of direct forms of market penetration in cash-hungry governments of poor countries via direct foreign investment, either by licensing with a domestic monopoly, joint ventures, or other strategic partnering with domestic companies (World Tobacco File 1998).

Box 8.2: **Impact of WTO entry on China**

Directly linked to the business opportunities offered by global trade liberalization, trans-national tobacco companies are anxiously awaiting further opening of the Chinese market. Due to China's long-standing restrictions on tobacco imports and exports, the dependency of China's tobacco industry on foreign trade has been minimal. Between 1995 and 1999 China's total imports and exports of leaf tobacco was only about 4.5 per cent of the domestic purchases on average, and total cigarette imports and exports made up a mere 0.8 per cent of domestic output on average.

As a result of its entry into the WTO, the Chinese domestic tobacco market must open up to foreign competition. With the industry's limited export capacity, the primary impact will be the shrinking domestic market share of practically all tobacco products produced under the monopoly. Cigarettes offer one example. China began to slash import duties on cigarettes in 1997 from a high of 150 per cent. In 1999, the rate fell to 36 per cent. Meanwhile, China's consolidated tax on imported cigarettes dropped to 218 per cent in 1999, down 26 per cent compared with 1997. The Chinese government has committed itself to a large-margin cut of the average tariff on all imported commodities, a high tariff on cigarettes violates that promise. Consequently, the Chinese government will continue to reduce the import duty on cigarettes. If the rate drops to the average for all imports, that is 15 per cent in the year 2000, one packet of imported cigarettes that sells for US$1.33 now (Marlboro and 555 brands) will sell for US$0.24–0.36 less after the reduction. This will greatly enhance the competitiveness of imported cigarettes on the Chinese market. Most of the adverse effects of cigarette imports on the domestic market after China's entry will not come from tariff reduction, but from the relaxation of non-tariff barriers. Permitted a long transition period, China's tobacco industry must gradually relax and finally abolish the quota and license controls that are now in force. Inevitably a large influx of foreign cigarettes will result.

In the absence of strong tobacco control policies in China, we can expect that trade liberalization will lead to more and better tobacco advertising, as well as more competition leading to lower prices. As a result, tobacco consumption is China could increase beyond its already catastrophic rates.

Source: Zhonggou 2000

Other aspects

The globalization of the tobacco pandemic is not limited to international trade and investment. Numerous other aspects of the tobacco epidemic are being fuelled by processes and practices that transcend national boundaries (Joosens 1999). For example, an estimated 355 billion cigarettes (33 per cent of the world market for exported cigarettes) are smuggled each year in order to avoid taxes. As one authority has noted, cigarette smuggling is now so widespread and well organized that it poses a serious threat to both public health and government treasuries, which are losing thousands of millions of dollars in revenue (Joosens 1999). Smuggled cigarettes are sold at below-market price, making top international western brands available to young people in developing countries, thereby increasing consumption and undermining efforts to keep children from smoking.

Trans-national tobacco marketing, advertising, and sponsorship also contributes to the global spread of tobacco use through worldwide media, such as cable and satellite television, the Internet and sponsorship of worldwide sports and entertainment events. Studies show that teenagers consume the cigarettes that most dominate sports sponsorship, while elementary children were most aware of the cigarette brands that are most frequently associated with sponsored sporting events on television (Ledwith 1984). These studies demonstrate that television sports sponsorship by tobacco manufacturers acts as cigarette advertising to children and therefore circumvents national laws banning cigarette advertisements on televisions.

As the vector of the tobacco epidemic, the tobacco industry is well aware of the characteristics of globalization and is attempting to manipulate globalization trends in its favour. Recently released documents of the multi-national tobacco industry concretely evidence that the industry 'plans, develops and operates its markets on a global scale' (Yach and Bettcher 2000). Further, a review of recent industry publications demonstrates that the industry looks towards the creation of new global brands and a global smoker as one way of overcoming markets which have thus far resisted the tobacco industry's onslaught (Crescenti 1998):

> [G]lobalisation has its limits. In India, for instance, around 80 per cent of the population uses traditional tobacco products such as bidis or chewing tobacco. . . For how long will these markets resist the attraction of global trends? In one or two generations, the sons and the grandsons of today's Indians may not want to smoke bidis or chew pan masala. . . Global brands are one way to accelerate this process.

In other words, industry strategists are encouraging the homogenization of the tobacco industry and the creation of a new global shared culture enshrined in the concept of a global smoker.

The global response

The globalization of the tobacco epidemic has critical policy implications. Low- and middle-income countries seeking to limit the impact of the global assault by trans-national tobacco corporations need to adopt and implement comprehensive tobacco control policies, including increasing the prices of tobacco products and restricting tobacco advertising and sponsorship. At the same time, the populations of industrialized countries remain at risk unless national tobacco control programmes are strengthened and reinforced. Moreover, the globalization of the tobacco pandemic 'restricts the capacity of countries to unilaterally control tobacco within their sovereign borders' (Taylor 1996). All trans-national tobacco control issues – including trade, smuggling, advertising and sponsorship, prices and taxes, control of toxic substances, and tobacco package design and labelling – require multilateral co-operation and effective action at the global level.

As Yach and Bettcher explain the combination of the tobacco industry's worth and powerful long-standing linkages to governments and a range of organs of civil society makes progress towards effective tobacco control, nationally and internationally, a difficult process. In contrast to the massive size of the challenge, global tobacco control has, until recently, lacked sustained global leadership, been severely underfunded and wanted for strategic direction (Yach and Bettcher 2000). However, the use of several governance mechanisms has created a platform for meaningful global action against the tobacco epidemic. These mechanisms include increased tobacco litigation: international leadership and global multi-sectoral co-operation; international law making; aggressive advocacy campaigns; and multiple new information tactics which reach out to civil society. Together, these mechanisms have extended the reach of the tobacco control message and are working to dramatically alter the tobacco governing structures.

Global governance

The concept of global governance expands the political space for members of the public health community to work in and provides numerous traditional and non-traditional structures with which they can expand their reach in promoting health issues. Global governance refers to the culmination of all spheres of authority (legal and social) at all levels of human activity that amount to systems of rules in which goals are pursued through the exercise of power (Rosenau 1997). The processes and mechanisms of global governance are diverse, as are the actors and structures that participate within them.

Modern societies emerge from a plurality of controlling actors. While national governments and the United Nations (UN) are central actors in the conduct of governance, they do not represent the whole picture. In addition to nation states, political actors also include international institutions, governmental organizations, and various non-state actors, regimes, values, and rules. These actors may be located at the local, provincial, national, trans-national, international, or global level. Exploring governance on the global scale does not require an exclusive focus on the agents and structures that are global in scope. In an ever-more globalized and interdependent world, boundaries become blurred and events which occur on one level may have consequences for what occurs at every other level (Rosenau 1997:10). The concept of global governance in international relations is a response to the perception that the nature of world politics has shifted, conceptualizing the world political community as a single space in which the boundaries between interstate relations and the nation state have become eroded (Lee and Dodgson 2000). In this context while the nation state remains the most important actor in world politics, the emerging structures of international governance to manage an increasingly globalized political space cannot be overlooked.

The various groups and organizations making up the public health community represent non-state actors with credible political influence in world politics. As a network of professionals with recognized expertise and competence in the area of human health, the public health community has an authoritative claim to policy-relevant knowledge within the domain of health and can govern societal behaviour through the dissemination of its knowledge. Moreover, public health activists can work to ensure that global health governance is marked by transparency, accountability, and incentives that promote public well-being (WHO 1998).

States identify their interests and recognize the latitude of action deemed appropriate in specific issue-areas through the manner in which problems are understood by policy makers (Haas 1992). Due to the insidious and uncertain nature of current health threats (such as tobacco), policy makers, unfamiliar with the evidence surrounding specific issues, are forced to turn to the public health experts for information and advice on the technical issues surrounding health policy. The public health community exercises an important dimension of political power by gathering scientific evidence, assessing risk, articulating the cause-and-effect relationships of complex public health problems, helping states identify their interests, framing the health issues for collective debate, proposing specific policies, and identifying salient points for negotiation.

The FCTC offers an example of the public health community exercising this power to influence international policy making. By gathering evidence and articulating the trans-national elements of the global tobacco epidemic, the public health community has provided a strong and convincing case that global co-operation is needed to curb the public health catastrophe caused by tobacco. It will be up to the public health community to continue to demonstrate that it is capable of linking public health evidence to effective policy options which will redefine state interests and positions in support of effective tobacco control.

As the definition of governance insinuates, international policy co-ordination is not in itself enough to accomplish the public health community's goals. Risk factors associated with ill health, such as tobacco, are often related to individual and societal choices in lifestyle which can not be governed through legislation alone. The public health community must enhance population health literacy and promote healthy choices and behaviours. The public health community is well placed within societies to identify and manipulate non-state levers of power, institutions, and modes of action to change lifestyles and consumer habits that would improve the overall health of the public.

Tobacco control offers an especially practical example of the need for public health professionals to go beyond policy. The adoption and entry into force of the FCTC will not mark the final victory in the tobacco control campaign. Even if all states adhere to the convention, ultimate public health success can only be recognized if the burden of disease caused by tobacco is reduced to zero. This can only happen if the health dangers linked to tobacco become part of the public consciousness. It has, therefore, been crucial that the FCTC process act as a launching pad to raise public awareness and change social behaviour towards tobacco. Throughout the FCTC process, public health advocates have been effective in reaching out to all levels of human interaction to elicit responses from regional, national, and international institutions and actors.

In the twenty-first century, public health professionals need new solutions to address the global factors affecting human health. The concept of governance offers a new way of thinking about the international system and the public health community's role in it. Most importantly, it offers a framework in which public health professionals can develop effective strategies for promoting global public health.

Litigation

Litigation against the tobacco industry and the public release of secret industry documents fundamentally reframed the global tobacco debate and have lent essential support to policy makers and advocates worldwide. Courts now represent a governing mechanism to hold the tobacco industry liable for the marketing and selling of deadly products.

Despite the statistics provided by public health professionals, between 1950 and 1998 the tobacco industry 'enjoyed a record of success in civil litigation unique to almost any industry, never paying one cent in settlements or awards for any injuries claimed by cigarette smokers in their civil lawsuits' (Hatfield 1996). This all changed in 1998, when tobacco companies agreed to a settlement – unprecedented in terms of monetary relief, injunctive requirements, and disclosure of internal tobacco company documents (Ciresi *et al.* 1999). The settlement in the state of Minnesota was quickly followed by a second major settlement which forced the industry to pay US$264 billion over a period of 25 years to 46 of the states of the USA to compensate for tobacco-related health costs (Settlement Agreement 1998). The key to this turn-around in litigation was the forced release of approximately thirty-five million pages of internal industry documents (US Supreme Court 1998). These documents revealed that the industry knew for over four decades that smoking tobacco caused cancer, that they were aware of the addictive nature of nicotine, and that they manipulated cigarette content to increase addiction. The documents also outline a well-thought-out and followed-through strategy to cover up this information, target vulnerable populations including youth and women, and undermine tobacco control efforts. The information contained in the millions of tobacco industry documents and the preliminary victories against the tobacco industry opened the flood gates for future tobacco litigation in the USA.

Since more information has been disclosed about the activities of the tobacco industry 'policy makers, programme personnel, and researchers' have focused on the tobacco industry as the 'underlying cause' of the tobacco epidemic (Cohen *et al.* 1999). At the last count some type of litigation is under way in at least 15 countries, ranging from personal class action litigation in Australia to health care recovery in Canada to public interest petitions in India. In addition, recent lawsuits filed have charged the tobacco industry with tobacco smuggling. In December 1999, the Canadian government filed a lawsuit under the Racketeer Influenced and Corrupt Organization Act in the US federal court. The government claimed that various RJ Reynolds tobacco companies and others defrauded the Canadian people by conspiring to smuggle tobacco into Canada. In November 2000, the European Commission, the executive arm of the EU, also filed suit against the two biggest American cigarette makers, Philip Morris and RJ Reynolds, accusing them of cigarette smuggling and asking for financial compensation for lost revenue and injunctive relief in order to prevent future smuggling (Schreyer 2000). In 1997, it was estimated that the European Community lost €5 billion every year as a result of cigarette smuggling and the losses have increased over the years (European Parliament 1997). The United Kingdom Customs and Excise Office have estimated that in the UK alone in 1999 losses were £2.5 billion or €4 billion (BBC Money Programme 2001)

Global litigation against the tobacco industry is being forwarded through international consultations and conferences. At the International Conference on Tobacco Control Law, hosted by the Government of India in New Delhi, several recommendations were made to facilitate international litigation. These recommendations included preventing double standards where multi-national companies exercise a higher degree of care in their home countries than when they operate abroad by including a provision allowing the use of the substantive laws of the home country if they are stricter than those in the country of harm; adopting the doctrine of enterprise liability to make trans-national tobacco companies liable for harm committed by their subsidiaries; and encouraging the sharing of information through the establishment of a tobacco litigation website (Global Tobacco Control Law 2000).

Global leadership in tobacco control and multi-sectoral collaboration

Global tobacco control received a major boost in 1998 when Gro Harlem Brundtland took over as Director General of the WHO. The new WHO Director General showed global leadership and support for tobacco control through the creation of the Tobacco Free Initiative as one of three central cabinet projects. The Tobacco Free Initiative provides an opportunity to create a global platform for meaningful action against the tobacco industry. Four priority areas that the Tobacco Free Initiative emphasizes are: (1) global information management, (2) development of nationally and locally grounded action, (3) the establishment of strong and effective partnerships, and (4) global regulation, legal instruments, and foreign policy. The WHO FCTC is the cornerstone of the Tobacco Free Initiative's efforts to control the global rise and spread to the tobacco epidemic through the promotion of national action and international co-operation (Yach and Bettcher 2000).

Recognizing that it does not have the institutional expertise to single-handedly address all the issues involved in tobacco control, the WHO has initiated global multi-sectoral co-operation on tobacco control. A strong network of partners, each with its own unique and complementary role in tobacco control, is solidifying the evidence base in support of global tobacco regulation and developing new mechanisms to implement tobacco control policies. In April 1999 the UN's Administrative Committee on Co-ordination (ACC), at the request of the WHO Director General and with support of UN Secretary General Kofi Annan, agreed that an *ad hoc* Inter-Agency Task Force on Tobacco Control (under the WHO's leadership) would replace the former UN focal point which had been situated within the UN Conference on Trade and Development (UNCTAD). Fifteen UN organizations, as well as the World Bank, the International Monetary Fund, and the WTO, are participating in the ongoing work of the task force which is significantly expanding the horizons for multi-sectoral collaboration across the UN. Since the establishment of the task force, new areas of co-operation have emerged, and prospects for future partnerships exist in a number of areas including the economics of tobacco control (lead agency the World Bank), world tobacco supply, demand, and trade by 2010 (lead agency the Food and Agricultural Organization), employment effects of tobacco control (lead agency the International Labour Organization), and environmental tobacco smoke (prospective collaborating partners include WHO, the International Civil Aviation Organization, the UN Environmental Programme, and UNICEF) (UNCTAD 2000).

As a result of these enhanced global efforts, effective multi-sectoral collaboration on the global scale has taken place between the WHO and the World Bank. The production and consumption of tobacco has an impact on the social and economic resources in both developed and developing countries. However, until recently these aspects have received little global attention. The World Bank, in collaboration with the WHO, released a report in 1999 which addressed the concerns raised by policy makers about the impact of tobacco control policies on economies (World Bank 1999). Based on numerous economic studies conducted by researchers at the World Bank and others, the report encourages governments to adopt a multi-pronged strategy which is tailored to the conditions within their respective country. In particular, the World Bank found that demand reduction strategies, such as tax increases, promotion bans, warning labels, restrictions on public smoking, and widened access to nicotine replacement therapies and other cessation therapies, were the most effective in the short term. The World Bank also urged other international agencies to join in the global campaign against tobacco by reviewing their policies, sponsoring research, addressing cross border issues, such as smuggling, and supporting the FCTC.

The FCTC process has also sparked multi-sectoral co-operation on the national level. Countries as diverse as Brazil, Thailand, and the USA have established formal multi-sectoral committees to prepare for the FCTC negotiations. In other countries, such as China, interministerial consultations are occurring on a regular basis. Formal and informal committees such as these are giving different ministries the opportunity, perhaps for the first time, to discuss and address the domestic burden of tobacco (Taylor 2000).

Dr Brundtland's powerful leadership in tobacco control is acting as an umbrella under which countries feel safe to speak out clearly(Yach and Bettcher 2000). During the Tobacco Free Initiative's initial two years of work it received demands for stronger action from governments who felt powerless in the face of tobacco industry pressure. New opportunities have, therefore, been created for senior legislators to share their experience and to hear that their problems are not unique. What has emerged is a stronger sense of global solidarity concerning the need for joint action between countries in diverse regions and at different levels of development.

The Framework Convention on Tobacco Control

Globalization is changing the shape of the structures of governance. Since nations are increasingly unable to maintain a firm hold on the economic and social conditions in their countries, states are increasingly developing international regulations, either at the global or regional level. At the international level these regulatory frameworks take the form of international conventions, which require the voluntary ratification of the contracting states. This new world order characterized by globalization will be increasingly characterized by four groups of regulations: world regulations as contained in international regulations; regional regulations, for example those of the EU, which may go beyond the model of international conventions; conventional national regulations; and sub-national regulations, such as the laws of states or provinces within a federated system (Basedow 2000). It is important to point out however, that to claim that international law should be developed more fully to regulate globalization more efficiently is not to imply an end to the role of states. On the contrary, international law is voluntarily created by states. Within this context not everything can or should be dealt with at the global level (Stern 2000). As outlined above, the future global regulatory framework will be comprised of complementary sub-national, national, regional, and international components. It is within this context that the FCTC fits into a global system of governance, which will be part of an integrated regulatory system comprised of local, national, regional, and global norms.

The framework convention–protocol approach has been used frequently and, at times, successfully to address a wide realm of international concerns, including environmental, arms control, and human rights issues (Taylor 1996).

The term framework convention does not have a particular technical meaning in international law. It is used to describe a variety of legal agreements which establish a general system of governance for an issue or area, such as global tobacco control (Bodansky 1999). Framework conventions, unlike more comprehensive forms of treaties, do not attempt to resolve all significant issues in a single document. Rather, framework conventions divide the negotiation of separate issues into separate agreements. States first adopt a framework convention which creates an institutional forum in which states can co-operate and negotiate for the conclusion of separate protocols containing detailed substantive obligations or added institutional commitments. The framework convention–protocol approach is, in essence, a 'dynamic and incremental process of global law-making.' (Taylor and Romer 1996).

The development and implementation of recent framework conventions have been closely linked to the accumulation of scientific evidence and assessment of trans-boundary risk. In particular, scientific evidence has been at the core of recent international environmental agreements, including the Framework Convention on Climate Change, the Vienna Convention for the Protection of the Ozone Layer, the Montreal Protocol, and the Bio-Diversity Convention. Scientific communities have been important actors, gathering and presenting the empirical evidence needed to support the development and ratification of these international conventions and protocols.

The FCTC is being developed as a scientific, evidence-based approach to global tobacco control (Taylor and Bettcher 2000). As the primary specialized agency addressing health matters, the WHO has the legal authority to serve as a platform for the development of binding treaties that potentially address all aspects of tobacco control, national and trans-national, as long as advancing human health is the primary objective of such agreements. It is within this context and within the institutional framework of the WHO that the public health community has been most effective in reaching states with the scientific evidence surrounding the global tobacco epidemic.

In order to consolidate the scientific foundation for the WHO convention and possible protocols, the WHO member states established in World Health Assembly Resolution WHA 52.18 the Working Group on the WHO FCTC. The mission of this intergovernmental technical body was to prepare proposed draft elements of the FCTC and to submit a report to the 53rd World Health Assembly, the governing body of the WHO. The working group provided an unprecedented opportunity to highlight tobacco control and educate and inform political leaders of the economic and health consequences of tobacco. The two meetings of the FCTC Working Group were attended by participants from a wide range of sectors and included representatives from 153 countries (representing 95 per cent of the world's population) and the European Community, as well as observers from the Holy See, Palestine, organizations of the UN system, and other intergovernmental organizations and non-governmental organizations (NGOs).

At its first meeting in October 1999, the working group agreed that substantive tobacco control obligations should focus principally on empirically established demand reduction strategies, as emphasized in the World Bank report, *Curbing the epidemic: governments and the economics of tobacco control* (World Bank 1999). Hence, the working group stressed that the WHO convention and possible protocols should promote global agreement and co-operation on the primary interventions on which there is overwhelming empirical support, including tobacco taxes and prices, advertising and promotion, mass media and counter-advertising, warning labels, clean air policies, and treatment of tobacco dependence.

At its second session in March 2000, the working group prepared a final report for the 53rd World Health Assembly which contained 'proposed draft elements'. The 'proposed draft elements' document was forwarded to the first session of the Intergovernmental Negotiating Body, the political body established by the WHO's member states to negotiate the FCTC (WHO 2000a). The draft elements resembled an international treaty on tobacco control, including objectives, guiding principles, obligations, institutions, implementation, and the development of the convention and final clauses. However, the elements were not a draft treaty in that they did not reflect the final political negotiating positions of member states. Instead, the elements offered a menu of possible options of those legal provisions which might be included in the FCTC or its protocols. On the first day of negotiations, however, the WHO member states agreed to use the draft elements as a reference document for initiating negotiations. The overwhelming acceptance of the draft elements as a basis to begin negotiations represented a first step forward in the public health community's quest to institutionalize its tobacco control evidence and policy proposals through binding treaty text.

The evidence provided by the public health community, as well as traditional state interests and power distribution, will define or redefine states' interests and positions on specific tobacco control issues which will eventually lead to a new global regime on tobacco. In the end, the negotiation of the FCTC and related protocols will depend on the prerogative of sovereign states. Most likely, governments will not be prepared to accept all the suggestions put forward by the public health community at the start of the FCTC negotiations. However, the framework convention–protocol approach allows for the incremental development of an international legal regime for global tobacco control. More issues could be appended, even after the ratification of the FCTC and initial protocol agreements. The FCTC process, even after ratification, will continue to provide a global instrument for public health professionals to distribute their evidence to governments and to get this evidence incorporated into binding agreements.

Advocacy

Tobacco control has traditionally been unable to compete with the tobacco companies' power to influence the behaviour of millions. Philip Morris's massive investments in marketing over the last 40 years recently resulted in Advertising Age provocatively naming Marlboro Man the number one advertising icon of the century. As explained in the accompanying text '[The Marlboro Man is] the most powerful – an in some quarters, most hated – brand image of the century' (Anonymous 1999). In contrast to the powerful Marlboro icon, the humble and well recognized no smoking sign has much less power to influence people's behaviour. Unlike the public health community, the tobacco industry does not speak the language of science and economics. Instead, it speaks the language of images, music, fun, and freedom to sell a product that kills half of its regular users.

With the FCTC leading the way, public health professionals have been forced to become much more aggressive in advocating the dangers associated with tobacco. In 1999, the WHO launched the global advocacy campaign entitled 'Tobacco Kills – Don't be Duped' (Box 8.3) which aimed to raise awareness and counter the global marketing practices of the tobacco industry which lures customers, especially young people, through sponsorship, advertising and glamorization of tobacco in films, music, art, and sports. The 'Don't be Duped' campaign sought to move tobacco control issues to the top end of national and international political agendas and to the centre of national public health debates. In doing so, the campaign sought out new language, a new idiom, and a new sense of purpose and direction for tobacco control. In contrast to the traditional no smoking sign, the symbol of the 'Don't be Duped' campaign was an image of two Marlboro cowboys riding into the sunset with one confiding in the other that he has cancer.

The campaign engaged and supported nationally based social entrepreneurs and change agents from the media, the NGO community, health professionals, or the private sector in target countries. Change agents were chosen based on their demonstrated interest in tobacco control, access to their own networks and position to influence policy in their own areas of focus. Workshops in media advocacy were organized with these change agents to mobilize opinion, as well as to support policy change and eventual ratification of the FCTC.

The 'Don't be Duped' campaign, originally launched in 16 countries in November 1999, culminated in heightened activity and policy announcements in several WHO member states on World No Tobacco Day 2000. In Pakistan, Imran Khan, former

Box 8.3: 'Tobacco Kills—Don't be Duped': towards a global platform to counter deception in public health

The political, social, and economic commitment and will to circumscribe, if not altogether prevent tobacco companies' domination of the 'health information market place' and its devastating effects on global health depends greatly on the effective development of a new health communication platform.

The 'Tobacco Kills – Don't be Duped' global media and NGO advocacy campaign seeks to plough the policy arena for the FCTC as WHO's 191 Member states negotiate the world's first public health treaty.

Funded by the United Nations Foundation (UNF), the campaign is based on the premise that at least five key constituents – media, NGOs, health professionals, the private sector, and ministries of health – have to mix and match their efforts for robust policy initiatives to emerge and take root. While the health sector is the convenor of the issue, unfolding in the context of the FCTC, the campaign seeks to activate all those areas of governance that have a direct impact on public health. The accuracy of the health debate sought by the campaign is leading health ministries to interface with ministries of trade, labour, finance, agriculture, and social services.

Thailand, China, the Philippines, India, Pakistan, Iran, Switzerland, Mali, South Africa, Zimbabwe, Germany, Ukraine, Venezuela, Brazil, and Norway make up the first group of countries where the campaign is active. Some of these countries have mobilized their own funds. The logic of 'Don't be Duped', however, has taken root beyond. The recent WHO Expert Committee on Tobacco Industry document has recommended that the logic of the campaign be extended to all WHO member states, especially to monitor tobacco company activities.

captain of the Pakistan cricket team, called on international sport – both players and organizations – to stop accepting sponsorship from tobacco companies. In Thailand, 10 000 people marched and sang anti-tobacco songs, while Dr Brundtland commended the king for his contribution to tobacco control. In India, the first tobacco website in Hindi was launched and various cities held screening examinations for smokers. In the Philippines, a mock parliament, dubbed the Children and Tobacco Congress and attended by over 200 children, passed a resolution asking the real congress to pass laws regulating the manufacture, sale, and marketing of cigarettes. In Mauritius, two NGOs announced their decision to request British American Tobacco, the sole manufacturer of cigarettes in the country, for compensation relating to the cost of treating diseases caused by tobacco. Legislation was announced in Brazil, South Africa, Lebanon, the EU, Malaysia, and Switzerland. These activities represent only a small handful of the global activities that took place on 31 May 2000.

Non-governmental organizations have also been effective in advocating the FCTC. The Framework Convention Alliance joins together over 60 non-governmental organizations, including many public health organizations, in support of global tobacco control. The alliance was formed out of the needs to enhance communication amongst groups already working around the FCTC process and for a more systematic outreach to NGOs not yet engaged in the process, particularly smaller NGOs in developing countries. Throughout the first session of the Intergovernmental Negotiating Body, the alliance held lunch time seminars on various technical aspects of the convention. In addition, the alliance distributed a bulletin each day to all delegates which highlighted a different area of interest to the FCTC and reported on the previous day's proceedings. Alliance members also placed the 'death clock,' which records a death caused by tobacco every eight seconds, just outside the negotiating room. Throughout the week the clock approached four million deaths caused by tobacco since the FCTC process began.

Public hearings

Another historic move in global tobacco governance occurred when the WHO hosted its first ever public hearings on the FCTC. In October 2000, all interested parties, including the tobacco industry, were invited to present their views before the WHO member states embarked on the negotiation of the convention. The WHO received 514 submissions, which were immediately made accessible for public scrutiny on the WHO's website. The hearings were effective in mobilizing public health organizations throughout the world to voice their support for global tobacco control. Throughout the two days of testimonies, over 90 public health groups took the floor. Speakers from the public health institutions and organizations expressed extreme concern about the impact of tobacco use on current and future health, especially in developing countries. They also argued that clear differences remained between their public health goals and the objectives of tobacco companies and that "*any participation by the tobacco companies in the negotiation and drafting of the FCTC should be categorically excluded from consideration by WHO member states*" (WHO 2000b). In addition, public health advocates argued against industry claims that environmental tobacco smoke or passive smoking was merely an annoyance to non-smokers and argued that major health concerns linked to passive smoking should be specifically addressed in the FCTC.

The FCTC public hearings were widely reported in the world's press and helped to intensify the tobacco control debate. Although tobacco companies have been quoted as admitting the addictive and deadly effects of their products in the USA, the public hearings provided the first truly global forum for these declarations.

The World Health Organization industry inquiry

The WHO also reached a global audience through its inquiry into tobacco company strategies to undermine its tobacco control activities. The release of the report resulted in worldwide media attention which intensified the tobacco control discourse and further discredited tobacco companies' efforts to recast their image as a responsible industry.

In the summer of 1999 the Tobacco Free Initiative began gathering evidence which suggested that WHO global tobacco control policies may have been affected by tobacco company practices aimed at influencing funding, policy, and research priorities. Based on this emerging evidence, Dr Brundtland assembled a Committee of Independent International Experts to verify if those fears were justified and what, if any, was the extent of damage done to the organization's public health policies. On 2 August 2000, the Committees 260-page report was publicly released on the Internet.

The report showed, through irrefutable documentary evidence, that tobacco companies viewed the WHO as one of their leading enemies, and that they saw themselves in a battle against the WHO. The documents also showed that tobacco companies fought the WHO's tobacco control agenda by, among other things, staging events to divert attention from the public health issues raised by tobacco use, attempting to reduce budgets for scientific and policy activities carried out by the WHO, pitting other UN agencies against the WHO, seeking to convince developing countries that the WHO's tobacco control programme was a 'First World' agenda carried out at the expense of the developing world, distorting the results of important scientific studies on tobacco, and discrediting the WHO as an institution (WHO 2000c).

The committee concluded that the tobacco companies' activities slowed and undermined effective tobacco control programmes around the world. Given the magnitude of the devastation wrought by tobacco use, the committee argued that it is reasonable to believe that the tobacco companies' subversion of the WHO's tobacco control activities has resulted in significant harm. Finally, the committee urged the WHO to take corrective and appropriate action and offered 58 recommendations aimed at protecting against the strategies employed by tobacco companies. Dr Brundtland accepted all recommendations and indicated that the WHO will work with other UN agencies, member states and NGOs to ensure that WHO processes are not subverted in the future.

Consultations and conferences

Numerous tobacco control consultations and conferences have been held since the World Health Assembly passed its resolution in 1999 paving the way for formal negotiations of the FCTC. These conferences have included the 11th World Conference on Tobacco or Health in Chicago, USA, the Conference on Tobacco Regulation in Oslo, Norway, the Conference on Tobacco Control Law in New Dehli, India, and the launch of the 'Don't be Duped' campaign in San Francisco, USA (opened by Jeffery Wigand whose story is the topic of the Hollywood movie *The insider*). These conferences have again brought media attention to tobacco control issues and have pulled policy makers on all levels into the FCTC process. For example, the Prime Minister of India, Shri Atal Bihari Vajpayee, opened the conference in New Delhi and spoke of the devastating effects of tobacco consumption in India and of his support for the FCTC (WHO 2000d). Informative technical conferences, which aim to pull in policy makers and public health professionals, will continue to be organized throughout the FCTC process.

Regaining control of dialogue is crucial in shifting public opinion with regard to tobacco. Activities such as the 'Don't be Duped' campaign and public hearings have been instrumental in framing and reframing key issues involved with tobacco. By signalling what is at stake, indicating who is responsible, and showing where solutions lie, tobacco control advocates have been able to confront the public with the facts about tobacco and influence policy outcomes. Moreover, the tobacco control community has been creative and aggressive in spreading their message. Multiple events in 2000, including World No Tobacco Day, the release of the WHO inquiry into tobacco company strategies to undermine its tobacco control activities, the FCTC public hearings, and the launch of formal negotiations resulted in worldwide press coverage and intensified public debate about tobacco control. By raising awareness, these activities are all working to shift the basic structures of global tobacco governance.

Concluding remarks

Global public health threats, such as the tobacco epidemic, pose new challenges to international health co-operation in the twenty-first century. While the public health communities' experience in catalysing new systems of global governance, which include the negotiation of binding regulatory frameworks such as conventions, is presently at a nascent phase of development, a wealth of experience already exists in other areas such as the environmental field. The notion of the 'tragedy of the commons' has led to a 'catastrophic overexploitation of common resources'. As part of addressing this global environmental crisis, over 120 multi-lateral environmental agreements had been negotiated by the early 1990s (Greene 1997). While many of these agreements have implications for public health, for instance the Ozone Treaty–Montreal Protocol and the Framework Convention on Climate Change–Kyoto Protocol, the public health community was not placed front and centre in shepherding the political process for their negotiation. However, as outlined in this chapter, with the evolution of new global initiatives to address the global health catastrophe posed by tobacco, the time has come to enhance the political profile of public health professionals and the public health community in pushing forward a global public health movement to address the tobacco epidemic.

While international regulatory and governance structures to confront public health problems have been historically quite weak, the global actions outlined in this chapter demonstrate a sea-change in international health co-operation. These actions include the negotiation of a legally binding treaty under the auspices of the WHO and the public health community, global public hearings to represent the voice of civil society, trans-national alliances of NGOs, innovative advocacy initiatives linking the local to the global spheres of political action, and international actions aimed at increasing the transparency and accountability of global trans-national actors, in particular the tobacco companies. Indeed, the FCTC has become more than a treaty, it is a public health movement (Subramaniam 1998).

As the UN agency responsible for global health co-operation, the WHO and its member states have recently taken important steps forward in tackling the tobacco threat in a more forthright fashion. For the first time in the 52-year history of the WHO, its member states have agreed unanimously to use the powers under Article 19 of WHO's constitution and negotiate a legally binding convention. As noted above, this also represents the first time that the public health community has been responsible for leading a treaty-making process. Therefore, for the first time in the history of public health the limelight is on us, and the onus is on public health professionals and other health groups to link into the various networks and processes outlined in this chapter, to initiate new initiatives, and to ensure that this historic process contributes to reducing the health impact of a totally preventable man-made epidemic.

The globalization of the tobacco epidemic is a tangible drawback of globalization. However, the public health community has the potential to use its solid scientific evidence base to strengthen the governance mechanisms for tobacco control, and in particular to develop an integrated regulatory framework which embraces sub-national/local, national, regional, and global norms. Global tobacco control represents a new era in global health co-operation. It is up to us as health professionals to ensure that new leadership for global tobacco control leads to concrete outcomes and a lasting impact in reducing the devastating death toll due to tobacco-related diseases.

References

Anonymous (1999) Advertising age. Top advertising icon. *The advertising century.* D. Klein and S. donaton, www.adage.com/century.

Basedow, J. (2000) The effects of globalization on private international law. In *Legal aspects of globalization*, ed. J. Basedow and T. Kono, p. 5. Kluwer Law International, The Hague.

Bodansky, D. (1999) *The framework convention protocol approach.* WHO, Geneva.

Chaloupka, F. and Corbett, M. (1998) Trade policy and tobacco: towards an optimal policy mix, In *The economics of tobacco control*, ed. I. Abedian van der Merwe R., Wilkins N. *et al.* Applied Fiscal Research Centre, Cape Town.

Chaloupka, F. and Warner, K. (1998) The economics of smoking. In *The handbook of health economics.* ed. A. J. Culyer and J. Newhouse. Elsevier, Amsterdam.

Ciresi M., Walburn, R., Sutton, T., *et al.* (1999) Decades of deceit: document discovery in the MINNESOTA tobacco litigation. *William Mitchell Law Review*, **25**(2).

Cohen, J. E., Ashley, M. J., Ferrence, R. *et al.* (1999) Institutional addiction to tobacco. *Tobacco Control*, **8**, 70–4.

Connoly, G. N. (1992) Worldwide expansion of the trans-national tobacco industry. *Journal of the National Cancer Institute Monographs*, **12**, 29–35.

Corrao, M. Guindon, E., Cokkinides, V. *et al.* (2000) Building the evidence base for global tobacco control. *Bulletin of the World Health Organization*, **78**, 884–90.

Crescenti, M. G. (1998) The new tobacco world. *Tobacco Journal International,* **3**, 51.

Doll, R. and Hill, A. B. (1954) The mortality of doctors in relation to their smoking habit; a preliminary report. *British Medical Journal,* **1**.

European Parliament. Committee of Inquiry into the Community transit system. Brussels, 1997.

Global Tobacco Control Law (2000) Towards a WHO framework convention on tobacco control, report of an international conference. *SEA-Tobacco–2 International Conference*, 7–9 January 2000, New Delhi,.

Greene, O. (1997) Environmental issues. In *The globalization of world politics*, ed. J. Baylis and S. Smith, Oxford University Press, Oxford.

Haas, P. (1992) Introduction: epistemic communities and international policy coordination. *International Organization*, **46**, 3.

Hatfield, C. (1996) The privilege doctrines – are they just another discovery tool utilized by the tobacco industry to conceal damaging information? *16 PACE Review*, **525**, 558.

Joosens, L. (1999) Improving public health through an international framework convention on tobacco control. FCTC technical briefing series, WHO/ncd/tfi/99. WHO, Geneva.

Ledwith, F. (1984) Does tobacco sport sponsorship on television act as advertising to children? *Health Education Journal*, **43**(4), 85–8.

Lee, K. and Dodgson, R. (2000) Globalization and cholera: implications for global governance. In *Global Governance: A Review of Multilateralism and International organizations*, **Vol. 6**, No. 2, pp. 227–8.

Murray, C. L. and Lopez, A. D. (ed.) (1996) The global burden of disease; a comprehensive assessment of mortality and disability from diseases, injuries and risk factors in 1990 and projected to 2020. Harvard School of Public Health, Cambridge, MA (on behalf of the WHO and the World Bank.)

Peto, R., Lopez, A. D., Boreham, J. et al. (1994) *Mortality from smoking in developed countries 1950–2000*. Oxford University Press. Oxford.

Peto, R. Lopez, A.D., Boreham, J. et al. (1998) Emerging tobacco hazards in China 1: retrospective proportional mortality study of one million deaths. *British Medical Journal*, **317**, 1411–22.

Roemer, R. (1993) Legislative action to combat the world tobacco epidemic, 2nd edn. WHO, Geneva.

Rosenau, J. (1997) *Along the domestic–foreign frontier: exploring governance in a turbulent world*, p. 145. Cambridge University Press, Cambridge.

Schreyer, M. (2000) Statement by EU Commissioner, November 6.

Settlement Agreement and Stipulation for Entry of Consent Judgement, State et al. Humphrey V, Philip Morris Inc., No C1–94–8565, 1998 WL 394331 (Min. Dist. Ct. May 8, 1998).

Stern, B. (2000) How to regulate globalization. In *The role of law in international poitics: essays in international relations and international law*, ed. M. Byers, pp. 266–7. Oxford University Press, Oxford.

Subramaniam, C. (1998) Advocacy for policy change. *NGO and Media Workshop*. Geneva.

Taylor, A. (1996) An international regulatory strategy of global tobacco control. *Yale Journal of International Law*, **21**(2), 257.

Taylor, A. (2000) The framework convention on tobacco control: the power of the process. *11th World Conference on Tobacco or Health*. Chicago.

Taylor, A. and Bettcher, D. (2000) WHO Framework convention on tobacco control: a global "good" for public health. *Bulletin of the World Health Organization,* **78**(7), 920–9.

Taylor, A., Chaloupka, F., Guindon, E. *et al.* (2000) *The impact of trade liberalization on tobacco consumption.* Oxford University Press, Oxford.

Taylor, A. and Romer, R. (1996) An international strategy for tobacco control, WHO/PSA/96.6. WHO, Geneva.

UNCTAD (2000) *Ad hoc* inter-agency task force on tobacco control. Report of the secretary-general, UNCTAD, substantive session of 2000. 5 July – 1 August, New York (ECOSOC Document E/2000/21).

US Department of Health and Human Services (1989) Reducing the health consequences of smoking: 25 Years of Progress. Report of the Surgeon General. Department of Health and Human Services, Rockville, Maryland.

US Department of Health and Human Services (1990) The health benefits of smoking cessation. Report of the Surgeon General. United States Department of Health and Human Services, Rockville, Maryland.

US Department of Health Services (1994) Preventing tobacco use among young people. Report of the Surgeon General. Office on Smoking and Health, US Government Printing Office, Washington.

US Environmental Protection Agency (1992) Respiratory health effects of passive smoking: lung cancer and other disorders. EPA fact sheet: respiratory health effects of passive smoking. January 1993, United States Environmental Protection Agency, Washington DC.

US Supreme Court (1998) Philip Morris Inc. v. Minnesota ex rel. Humphery, 118 s. Ct. 1384, www.tobaccoarchives.com and www.tobaccodocuments.org.

Vaughan, J., Collins, J., and Lee, K. (2000) Case study report: global analysis project on the political economy of tobacco control in low – and middle – income countries. School of Hygiene and Tropical Medicine, London.

World Bank (1999) Curbing the epidemic – governments and the economics of tobacco control. World Bank, Washington DC.

WHO (1998) Health for all in the 21st Century.

WHO (1999a) Tobacco free initiative consultation report, international consultation on environmental tobacco smoke and child health, unpublished document WHO/TFI/99.10. WHO, Geneva.

WHO (1999b) World Health Report. WHO, Geneva.

WHO (2000a) Proposed draft elements for a WHO framework convention on tobacco control: provisional texts with comments of the working group. 26th July, WHO, Geneva.

WHO (2000b) Public hearings on the framework convention on tobacco control. Document A/FCTC/INB1 INF.DOC/1.

WHO (2000c) Tobacco company strategies to undermine tobacco control activities at the World Health Organization. Report of the Committee of Experts on Tobacco Industry Documents. Tobacco Free Initiative, WHO, Geneva.

WHO (2000d) Speech available in global tobacco control law: towards a WHO framework convention on tobacco control. Report of an international conference, New Delhi.

World Tobacco File (1998). International Trade Publications Ltd, London.

Yach, D. and Bettcher, D. (2000) Globalization of tobacco industry influence and new global responses. *Tobacco Control*, **9**, 206–16.

Zhonggou, J. S. (2000) China's tobacco industry could get smoked by WTO entry. China Economic Times, May 10.

Chapter 9

Migration, equity, and health

Harry Minas

Population movements are the motor of history (Huntington 1996)

Introduction

Migration is a perennial fact of human history. Virtually all contemporary nations have been profoundly shaped by migration.

> For the fatherland of the English race we must look far away from England itself. In the fifth century after the birth of Christ, the one country which bore the name of England was what we now call Sleswick, a district in the heart of the peninsula which parts the Baltic from the Northern seas (Green 1992)

At other times, Romans, Normans and, more recently, Jews from eastern Europe and West Indians and South Asians from the British Commonwealth played their part in the formation of the country that now bears the name of England. During the sixth and seventh centuries the slow but massive south-western migration of the Slavs created the nations of the Balkans. During the seventeenth and eighteenth centuries the Empire of Vietnam gradually expanded southward. By the eighteenth century, the Vietnamese had populated all of present-day Vietnam from the Red River in the north to the Mekong Delta in the south, absorbing the former Cham Empire in central Vietnam and the south-eastern region of the Khmer (Cambodian) Empire around the Mekong. Between 1840 and 1920 more than 50 million people moved from Europe to North America (Kraut 1994). Australia, Canada, and New Zealand are relatively recent settler countries.

Forced migration has a similarly long history, even if the term 'ethnic cleansing' has only emerged at the end of the twentieth century. Since the fifteenth century approximately 40 million slaves were forcibly taken from Africa to work in the western hemisphere. In the two centuries following the Spanish Inquisition and the expulsion of Jews from the Iberian peninsula, there were more than one million refugees in Europe. After the Greek–Turkish war of the early 1920s, a population exchange occurred in which 1.2 million Greek Christians living in Turkey were resettled in Greece and 650 000 Turkish Muslims were moved from Greece to Turkey.

In the twentieth century, however, the nature of international migration changed in several important ways (Castles and Miller 1998). First, fragmentation of former empires into ever-smaller sovereign states, each with clearly demarcated borders and barriers to mobility, converted what would previously have been internal migrants into international migrants. Second, the determinants and mechanisms of migration are changing in response to a wide range of globalizing forces. These changes are extremely complex. In some cases, local conflicts that displace people have their roots in international trade, such as that in diamonds in West Africa. The increasingly global reach of information offers hope to many of a better life elsewhere. Taran (1999) has identified the ways in which certain features of economic globalization (such as structural adjustment, technological change, and the globalization of work, and trade liberalization) have had a direct impact on migration. Large numbers of people have experienced increased marginalization and exclusion in the form of unemployment or underemployment, reduced real earnings for those who are employed, erosion of job security, increasing poverty, reduced public services such as access to health care and education, and reduced social provision for the ill and the unemployed. Conversely, many of the strongest advocates of global movement of goods and services have fought hardest to block free movement of labour as they depend for their profits on the lower wages and poorer working conditions in less developed countries. Thus, in a period when it is easier than ever for the rich to travel the world, the poor face controls on international migration that are tighter than ever. The net effect of these changes can be seen from the change in the number of migrants (people living outside their country of birth), which was 75 million in 1965 and 120 million in 1990. This does, however, need to be kept in perspective. In 1981 India alone had 200 million internal migrants. The number of international arrivals of tourists per year increased from 69 million in 1960 to 450 million in 1990 (Zlotnik 1999).

Nonetheless, in 1965 there were 34 countries in which more than 15 per cent of the population were international migrants. By 1990, this number had grown to 52 countries. More countries have become destinations for international migrants, and the number of source countries has also increased. One in every 13 persons living in the west is an international migrant, with approximately two per cent of the global population (120 million) living outside their country of birth (Zlotnik 1999). Of these 55 per cent (65 million) are living in developing countries (Table 9.1).

Understanding migration

Migration is not an event. It is a complex and remarkably varied process (Fig. 9.1). People migrate because they can no longer tolerate living in the place where they were born, or because they have dreams of a place that is so much better that they will sometimes do anything it takes to get there. The journey may be a few hours by plane or may involve years of waiting in refugee camps and detention centres. For most people migration is an orderly and planned affair, marked by the bureaucratic tasks of filling in application forms, attending consular interviews, thinking about points systems and quotas for various categories of immigrants, dealing with travel or employment recruitment agents, and interminable waiting. For some it is a desperate flight in circumstances of great danger. Many thousands of people died at sea during the flight from Indochina in the late 1970s and early 1980s, because they were in

Table 9.1 Number of migrants by region

	1965 (millions)	1990 (millions)
North America	12.7	23.9
Western Europe	11.7	22.9
South-Central Asia	18.6	20.8
Western Asia	4.7	14.3
Sub-Saharan Africa	6.9	13.6
East & Southeast Asia	8.1	7.9
Latin America	5.9	7.5
Oceania	2.5	4.7
Northern Africa	1.0	2.0
Eastern Europe	2.8	2.0

Source: Zlotnik (1999), Table 1a, p. 47.

unseaworthy or overcrowded boats, because they got lost and ran out of food and water, or as a result of attacks by pirates in the South China Sea. In December 2000, 169 illegal immigrants, predominantly from the middle east, drowned in a storm at sea off the north coast of Australia. Fifty-eight young men, migrating illegally from southern China to Britain, were found dead on 18 June 2000 in an airtight container on the back of a Dutch truck in the English port of Dover.

Factors Influencing migrant flows

The factors that influence international migrant flows are complex and dynamic, and are intimately tied to broad political, social, and economic issues that are particularly important in poor countries. Most people who migrate would rather not have done so if they had reasonable access to the necessities of life – safety, food, shelter, freedom, and opportunity. The decision to migrate is rarely made lightly. People move because their current circumstances have become intolerable and/or because they see greater opportunities for themselves and their children elsewhere. In order to move, they must have access to the opportunity and the necessary resources. This means that it is rarely the poorest and the most vulnerable who migrate because they are least likely to be able to marshal the resources necessary to migrate and to establish themselves successfully in a new setting. Complex interactions between necessity, individual initiative, and opportunity remain the main determinants of migration.

War, civil disorder, natural disaster, poverty, and systematic infringements of human rights will continue to result in large numbers of migrants, refugees, and internally displaced people. Population growth and environmental degradation, including the consequences of climate change (Chapter 5) will result in massive movements of people, although most of these movements will be within countries rather than international migration. The scope for man-made disasters has increased

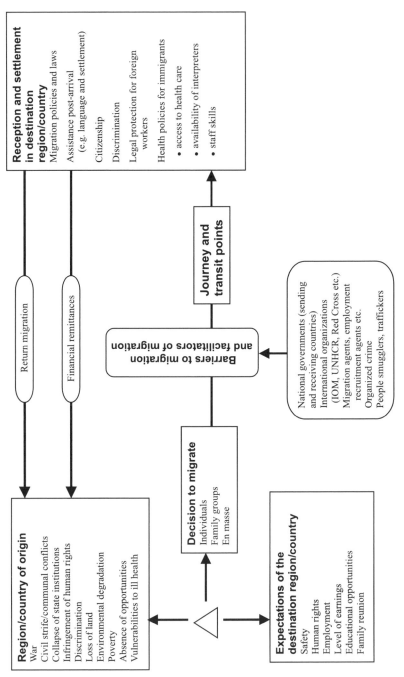

Figure 9.1 The complex nature of international migration

markedly, as illustrated by events at Chernobyl and Bhopal. The massive movement of people from rural regions to the mega-cities is already well under way.

Types of migration

Permanent settlement

For the traditional immigrant settler countries (the USA, Canada, Australia, New Zealand, and Israel) immigration was integral to their 'founding' and development as modern nations. They have continued to accept large numbers of immigrants, although intakes have fluctuated over recent decades. Developing countries predominate as the source countries for immigrants settling in Australia, Canada, and the USA (Freeman 1995). The UK, France, Portugal, and other former colonial powers experienced considerable immigration after the World War 2 that was driven by post-colonial obligations to the people of former colonies.

Temporary labour migration

> A world market for labour does not exist in the same way as it exists for goods and services. Most labour markets continue to be nationally regulated and only marginally accessible to outsiders, whether legal or illegal migrants or professional recruitment. Moving goods and services is infinitely easier than moving labour. Even a rapid and sustained expansion of the world economy is unlikely to significantly reduce the multiple barriers to the movement of labour. . . Extra-regional migration of all kinds is a small percentage of global labour movements. Most migration is of the country next door variety (Hirst and Thompson 1996)

In the post-war period, with reconstruction of economies and rapid industrial expansion, countries such as Germany and other European countries began to recruit large numbers of temporary labour immigrants. Prior to the economic collapse of the late 1990s, Hong Kong, Singapore, Japan, Malaysia, South Korea, and Taiwan greatly increased their intake of foreign workers, particularly from countries such as the Philippines and Indonesia. Following the economic downturn, many of these foreign workers were expelled. In countries such as the Philippines, the overseas employment of members of the Philippine population has developed into a national policy which is assessed mainly on two dimensions – job generation and foreign exchange remittances (Tomas 1999). Although the economic benefits are clear, the social costs – such as fragmented households, single-parent arrangements, and marital break-up – are less well understood.

The expanding middle classes in Asia, such as Malaysia, South Korea, and Singapore, rapidly increased their demand for foreign female domestic workers from Indonesia and the Philippines, until the currency crisis in the late 1990s. In 1994 there were 70 000 Filipina and Indonesian domestic workers in Malaysia. Various forms of mistreatment of these workers have been common, including failure to pay agreed salaries, sexual assault, and restriction of free movement encapsulated by the following quotation: 'Maria Rosa: See, they don't think we are human. We are like slaves to them. They take our sweat but they don't give us respect' (Chin 1997). Local newspapers carry regular discussions concerning the lack of labour rights for foreign domestic workers, their mistreatment and occasional murder, and suicides.

Many recent labour migration flows, particularly in Asia, have been predominantly of women. This is because of the increasing education of women and the loosening of restrictive social norms making migration possible, and also because of the desire of employers in receiving countries for low-paid workers who are, according to prevailing stereotypes, more easily controlled (Castles 1999). A source of increasing concern has been the trafficking of women for the sex industry, particularly of women from impoverished regions in underdeveloped countries or countries undergoing rapid and chaotic social and economic transitions, such as parts of the former Soviet Union. Exploitation of workers in unsafe working conditions, with very low rates of pay, affects women disproportionately. Domestic female workers, for example in Asia and the middle east, are particularly vulnerable to exploitation, abuse, and infringement of human rights. Undocumented and illegal migration makes it extremely difficult to gather data on such activities and working conditions, and virtually impossible to safeguard the rights of such immigrants. The weakness of sending countries in protecting the rights of their nationals who are labour migrants is very apparent.

Short-term migration by professionals is becoming increasingly common as part of the process of globalization, whether through employment by multi-national corporations that move their staff around the globe for varying periods or working with international organizations of various kinds.

Refugees/asylum seekers

Since the nineteenth century the dominant form of global political organization has been the nation state (see Chapter 2). It is important to distinguish the *territorial nation*, which may contain many ethnic groups (such as the English, Welsh, Scots, and Northern Irish in Britain, the many ethnic groups in Indonesia, etc.) and the ethnic nation, which is a community based on common descent. This may be a nation in search of a state, such as the Kurds and Palestinians. Multi-national (that is, multi-ethnic) states are the norm and claims to state legitimacy are based on civic assent rather than on descent. An ongoing task for many states is the development and consolidation of a common nationality by creating and fusing national identity with the political project of establishing or maintaining a state. Yugoslavia was one such effort that failed spectacularly. A more peaceful failure was the division of Czechoslovakia. States deal with ethnic pluralism (that is, the presence in the state of two or many nations or ethnic groups) in one of four ways (Keely 1996).

(1) The creation of a supranational identity that is separate from any of the constituent groups, a model followed by Indonesia in modern times.

(2) The creation of a national identity based on one dominant group, requiring other groups to conform to the dominant culture. This process may destroy other peoples as nations, along with their culture, language, history, identity, and, in extreme cases, their lives.

(3) A third method of dealing with the presence of multi-nationalism is 'ethnic cleansing.' This can be accomplished by population transfers (for example between Turkey and Greece following the Greek–Turkish war in the early 1920s) or between India and Pakistan after partition. It might be simple expulsion by violence – the expulsion of Moors and Jews from Spain in 1492, the Armenians by Turkey after World War 1, the Jews during World War 2, the Macedonians from Greece, and, more recently, the Albanian Kosovars. The ultimate form of ethnic cleansing is genocide.

(4) Finally, multi-nationalism can be handled by the creation of a federation, as in Canada, and until recently Yugoslavia, or a confederation as in Switzerland.

All of these patterns contain the possibility of conflict and violence.

A nation state may produce forced migration for three reasons.

(1) The state contains more than one nation.

(2) The populace disagrees about the structure of the state or the economy. Revolutions and their consolidation or failure produce refugees. There are innumerable examples in recent history of revolution and other forms of civil unrest producing refugees.

(3) The state fails as a functional organization with consequent social chaos. The characteristics of state failure include a lack of functioning government or an operative judicial system, failure of health and education systems and other basic social services, primitive internal markets and cessation of international trade, failure of organized agriculture and the mechanisms for distribution of food and other goods, and the collapse of banking and other financial institutions and services. Recent examples include Afghanistan, Somalia, Angola, Liberia, Rwanda, Sierra Leone, Kosovo, and East Timor. The causes of state failure can include withdrawal of external support from a weak state (with several recent examples following the end of the Cold War), corruption and incompetence, natural disaster, and dramatic changes in international market forces.

> The international response to refugee flows. . . is [also] founded in the nation-state system. Because people are supposed to be under the protection and normally within the boundaries of their state, any large, uncontrolled movement of people beyond their borders threatens international political stability. . .[T]he political basis for the international refugee regime is the protection of states and the international system of states that is threatened when states fail to fulfil their proper roles (Keely 1996)

There were, in 1998, approximately 13 million refugees worldwide, and a further 20 million people internally displaced in their own countries (US Committee for Refugees 1999). Although developed countries contribute most of the funding for refugee programs, the overwhelming majority of the world's refugees are in the world's poorest countries, which experience severe challenges because of their willingness to provide asylum to large numbers of refugees. An indicator of the challenges to poor countries in providing asylum to refugees is the ratio of the number of refugees to the population of the host country (US Committee for Refugees 1999) (Table 9.2).

Table 9.2 Ratio of refugees to host country population, 1998

Host country	Number of refugees	Ratio of refugee population to total population
Gaza Strip*	773,000	1:1
Jordan	1,463,800	1:3
West Bank*	555,000	1:3
Lebanon	368,300	1:11
Guinea	514,000	1:15
Yugoslavia	480,000	1:22
Liberia	120,000	1:23
Djibouti	23,000	1:30
Iran	1,931,000	1:33
Zambia	157,000	1:61
Sudan	360,000	1:79
Tanzania	329,000	1:93
Libya	28,000	1:100
United States	651,000	1:415
Germany	198,000	1:416
Canada	46,000	1:665
Russian Federation	206,500	1:711
United Kingdom	74,000	1:799
France	17,800	1:3,303
Japan	400	1:316,000

* Areas within Israeli occupied territories

The number of applications for asylum filed in European countries increased from 66 900 in 1983 to 694 000 in 1992, declined to 330 000 in 1994 and has remained at about that level (Zlotnik 1999). Asylum seekers and refugees are met with an increasingly 'frosty reception' (Castles 1999) in many countries, including those countries that have previously taken large numbers of refugees where there has been a sharp decline in willingness to accept refugees. For example, Germany, which had received the greatest number of refugees of any European country from 1983 to 1997, amended its Basic Law so as to reject claims for asylum by persons who had entered Germany through neighbouring countries considered safe under German asylum provisions. This resulted in a sharp decline in asylum claims filed in Germany.

Along with other western countries, and in response to perceived economic and cultural threats posed by large numbers of immigrants and refugees, the USA has applied more restrictive policies to migrants and asylum seekers (McBride 1999). Revisions in immigration and naturalization service procedures include 'expedited removal' procedures and stricter guidelines on deportation and detention. Australia has also taken a harsher approach to refugees and, particularly, to asylum seekers.

Many refugees and asylum seekers are victims of injury, brutality, rape, and deprivation of liberty, rights, and the necessities of life. Between 5 and 35 per cent of refugees have been subjected to state-sponsored torture.

The circumstances in which refugees live during flight and in refugee camps are such that malnutrition and disease (due to lack of clean water, sanitation, crowding) are the norm. Medical resources are either unavailable or very limited. Violence in refugee camps (including murder and rape) replaces the violence from which refugees have fled. Illegal return of refugees to the country of origin by the host country authorities (in contravention of the principle of 'non-refouillement') is becoming more common. Countries around the world are increasingly closing their doors to refugees. Many developed countries have implemented new requirements to limit or to prevent the entry of refugees (Marsella 1994). These include:

- stricter visa requirements for foreign nationals
- penalties for airlines that bring passengers without proper entry documents
- new eligibility requirements for asylum, stricter requirements for entry into countries of first asylum
- reductions in social and economic support rights and benefits (for example access to health care)
- prolonged periods of collective accommodation or administrative detention
- restricted quotas for refugees in immigration programs.

A new development as part of the international refugee regime in recent years is the introduction of temporary 'safe haven' programs, which may gradually replace the former sense of obligation to accept refugees as permanent settlers. Asylum seekers may be held in detention for years while their application for refugee status is processed, either in the country of first asylum or in the destination country for onshore asylum seekers.

Illegal/undocumented migration

Salt and Stein (1997) make a case for treating migration as a global business that has both legitimate and illegitimate components.

> The migration business is conceived as a system of institutionalised networks with complex profit and loss accounts, including a set of institutions, agents and individuals each of which stands to make a commercial gain (Salt and Stein 1997)

The core of the illegitimate business of migration is people trafficking.

> Organized transborder criminality of all kinds is currently thriving. This is the era of globalisation of crime, corresponding to the increase in global trade, personal mobility and high-tech communications. Traditional forms of trans-border organised crime such

as drug, weapons and motor vehicle smuggling and money laundering continue to exist. At the same time, however, many organizations involved in these activities have expanded their portfolio to include trafficking in migrants (Editorial 1996).

It is estimated that 200 000 Bangladeshi women have been trafficked to Pakistan in the past ten years. Twenty–thirty thousand Burmese women are estimated to be working as prostitutes in Thailand through forms of trafficking such as deceptive job advertisements, abduction, and sale of girls from hill tribes. At least 10 international crime syndicates are thought to be trafficking Thai women into Australia for the purpose of prostitution. More than 150 000 women, mostly from the Philippines and Thailand, work as prostitutes in Japan (Editorial 1997a).

Within country (rural–urban) migration

A focus on cross-border migration may obscure the magnitude of migration that takes place within countries and which may raise many similar issues.

In 1994, the 'floating population' of Beijing was 3.3 million (up from 1.3 million in 1988) and in Shanghai 3.3 million (from 2.1 million in 1988) representing 31 per cent and 25 per cent respectively of those two cities' populations. If these percentages are applied to China's total urban population of approximately 300 million, then the total size of the 'floating population' in Chinese cities is probably about 75–90 million people. Government officials cite a figure of 80 million. Mexican labour migration to the USA was, until the Chinese case, 'the largest sustained flow of migrant workers in the contemporary world' (Roberts 1997)

Roberts (1997) asserts that there are several similarities between the Chinese rural–urban labour migration and the undocumented migration of Mexicans to the USA.

(1) As is the case for migration in many developing countries, the migration is largely circular and not permanent. Migrants regularly return to their place of origin and maintain their ties to the land.

(2) There is in both cases a very large gap in the wages and standards of living between sending and receiving areas.

(3) There are restrictions preventing settlement of labour immigrants in both Chinese cities and in the USA. Enforcement of these regulations is often capricious creating much uncertainty as to the status of the immigrants since their labour is desired but their presence is not.

(4) Proximity between sending and receiving areas allows the process to be spontaneous rather than organized.

Return migration

Migration is, however, not a one-way process. The example of Senegal illustrates the dynamic nature of migration flows (Diatta and Mbow 1999). Because of its political stability and economic growth, Senegal was an important destination country in West African migration. In recent decades, continuing desertification and the economic impacts of globalization have changed Senegal from a country of immigration to one of emigration, with large numbers of migrants going to France, Côte D'Ivoire and Gabon. Senegal has initiated innovative programs that seek to increase the participation of Senegalese living abroad in the national social and economic development efforts. These programs have resulted in very large financial remittances ($US10 billion per year) to Senegal. These programs are linked with programmes intended to assist returning immigrants in re-integrating in Senegal and putting skills they have acquired abroad to productive use.

Other initiatives have sought to address the challenges arising from increasing international educational and occupational mobility. This has led to loss of highly qualified and skilled workers from poor countries in Africa, Asia, and elsewhere. This 'brain drain' has been substantial, with some 100 000 highly qualified Africans, nearly one-third of Africa's skilled workforce, working abroad, mainly in Western Europe and North America (10M International Organization for Migration, RQAN Return of Qualified African Nationals Programme Fact Sheet). The reasons for this massive movement of skilled workers are similar to the reasons for most migration – unattractive political, social, and economic conditions, low salaries with little hope of improvement, and attractive salaries and working and living conditions in western countries. Programs such as RQAN are beginning to have some effect in a number of regions in the world.

Conversely, international migration is of considerable economic significance to many developing countries because of the importance of net worker remittances. In the World Bank World Development Report for 1996 it was noted that net workers' remittances transferred to developing countries had increased from US$15 billion in 1980 to US$30 billion in 1994 (Table 9.3) (World Bank 1996). Remittances of money home by migrants constitute an important component of international financial flows and of the national incomes of a number of small states. Remittances rose form $3133 billion in 1970 to $30 401 billion in 1988 (Segal 1993, cited in Hirst and Thompson 1999).

Table 9.3 Net annual workers' remittances by country

	$US billion/year
Egypt	5.1
India	4.8
Mexico	3.7
Morocco	2.1
Pakistan	1.5
Jordan	1.1
Bangladesh	1.1
El Salvador	1.0

Source: World Bank, 1996

Table 9.4 Age at death, 1995–97. All Australians and indigenous Australians

	<50 years		50–64 years		65+ years	
	All Australians %	Indigenous %	All Australians %	Indigenous %	All Australians %	Indigenous %
Males	13.6	53.0	13.7	24.3	72.7	22.7
Females	7.6	41.7	9.2	20.5	83.3	31.8

Source: Australian Institute of Health and Welfare (2000)

Migration and health

Large-scale migration and colonization over the past several centuries has often had a devastating and remarkably sustained impact on the health of indigenous peoples. In Australia, at the end of the twentieth century, the epidemiology of disease among Aboriginal people is more like that of low-income countries than that of a relatively wealthy industrialized country. The life expectancy at birth of Aboriginal people is approximately 20 years less than that of the rest of the Australian population; 72.7 per cent of Australian males and 83.3 per cent of Australian females live beyond the age of 65 years, while only 22.7 per cent of Aboriginal males and 31.8 percent of Aboriginal females live beyond 65 years (Table 9.4; Australian Institute of Health and Welfare 2000). This dramatic difference in mortality is mirrored by equally disturbing figures concerning various forms of morbidity and disability.

The pattern of disease and mortality among immigrants is extremely varied, so much so that it is not useful to talk about immigrants as a homogeneous group. The health of immigrant groups is influenced by many factors, including the health risks to which they were exposed (and their access to health care) prior to and during the process of migration; the new health risks to which they are exposed during settlement in the new country; the stresses of migration and settlement, including poverty, unemployment, and discrimination; and their access to health care in the new country. There is the additional factor that migrants are generally subject to health screening and only those who are healthy are admitted into the new country. Table 9.5 (Australian Institute of Health and Welfare 2000) shows mortality differentials for the years 1996–1998 by birthplace, cause of death, and sex, for the Australian-born and for immigrants aged 15 years and over. It can be seen that the pattern of differences is quite complex and that for most causes of death the age standardized mortality ratios (SMRs) for the immigrant groups are significantly different to those for the Australian-born. It is generally the case that rates of disease among immigrant groups become more like those in the host population the longer the immigrant group has been living in the host country, that is the longer the immigrant group is exposed to the same health risks and benefits as the host population.

Immigrants are more likely to be poor and to have less access to effective health services than the native-born. This is particularly so for those who are unskilled and who do not speak the language of the host country. In 1997 there were 25.7 million foreign-born

Table 9.5 Health of immigrants in Australia: mortality differentials by birthplace, cause of death and sex, age 15 years and over, 1996–8

ICD-9-CM	Males					Females				
	Standardized mortality ratio (Australian-born = 1.0)					Standardized mortality ratio (Australian-born = 1.0)				
	Total	UK and Ireland	Other Europe	Asia	Other	Total	UK and Ireland	Other Europe	Asia	Other
Infectious	2,558	0.79*	1.01	1.39*	1.39*	1,742	0.84*	1.36*	1.52*	1.24*
AIDS	1,005	0.84*	0.76*	0.49*	1.44*	95	0.95	0.58*	1.32	1.61
Cancers	58,685	0.94*	0.90*	0.64*	0.84*	45,508	1.05*	0.85*	0.71*	0.94*
Lung	14,092	1.16*	1.07*	0.68*	0.91*	6,139	1.49*	0.66*	0.83*	0.95
Skin	2,489	0.42*	0.34*	0.10*	0.45*	1,326	0.63*	0.40*	0.10*	0.68*
Prostate	7,592	0.80*	0.64*	0.42*	0.83*	n.a.	n.a.	n.a.	n.a.	n.a.
Breast	n.a.	n.a.	n.a.	n.a.	n.a.	7,731	1.09*	0.86*	0.61*	1.05*
Cervix	n.a.	n.a.	n.a.	n.a.	n.a.	861	1.03	0.87*	1.23*	1.19*
Diabetes mellitus	4,340	0.83*	1.27*	1.18*	1.27*	4,183	0.76*	1.74*	1.54*	1.56*
Cardiovascular	76,319	0.88*	0.86*	0.61*	0.90*	79,851	0.87*	0.84*	0.70*	0.95*
Respiratory	18,980	0.95*	0.64*	0.58*	0.67*	16,462	1.03*	0.56*	0.58*	0.83*
Digestive	5,892	0.86*	0.84*	0.63*	0.71*	5,719	0.99	0.74*	0.65*	0.86*
Injury and Poisoning	15,631	0.89*	0.84*	0.58*	0.90*	6,393	1.05	0.96	0.94	1.04
Motor vehicle	3,663	0.79*	0.79*	0.69*	0.99	1,495	1.10	1.21*	1.20*	1.16*
Suicide	6,155	0.93*	0.74*	0.40*	0.79*	1,544	0.95	0.92	0.83*	0.97
Homicide	603	0.79*	1.53*	1.44*	1.63*	286	1.08	1.31	0.98	0.83
All causes	195,135	0.88*	0.82*	0.54*	0.79*	176,626	0.93*	0.81*	0.62*	0.86*

* Significantly different from 1.00 at the 5% level. (Rates that are significantly higher among immigrants than the Australian-born are shown in italics).
Source: Table 4.10, p. 205: Australian Institute of Health and Welfare (2000)

people in the USA (Table 9.6; US Census Bureau, 1999), constituting 9.7 per cent of the total US population. The largest group of foreign-born in 1997, those from Latin American countries, had the highest rate of poverty and the lowest rate of health-insurance coverage. Immigrants from Europe had poverty and health-insurance coverage rates very similar to those of the native-born population (Table 9.6).

Infectious diseases

Migration is closely linked to the incidence and spread of infectious diseases in a number of ways. The first is that the factors that contribute to the emergence of new infectious diseases, and to the failure to control existing, well-understood, infectious diseases, are very similar to the factors that contribute to migration. These include poverty; ecological degradation; rapid urbanization and overcrowding; breakdown of civil institutions, including public health measures; social and economic inequalities; failure to protect human rights, including access to health services, adequate housing, food, and safe drinking water; and natural and man-made disasters including war (Farmer 1996; Morse 1995). Global inequalities are expressed in massive disparities in effectiveness of disease control, resulting in major regional, and social class, differences in the incidence and prevalence of diseases.

The second is that the direction of migration is overwhelmingly from regions of high infectious disease prevalence to regions of low infectious disease prevalence. The movement of people between from high prevalence to low prevalence regions has been the historical impetus for the development of quarantine arrangements in fourteenth-century Europe, one of the oldest organized public health practices (Chapter 4) and more recent migration health-screening arrangements (Editorial 1997*b*, 1998). In recent times, health screening has been used also both as a tool for excluding potential immigrants who are considered undesirable by immigration authorities (such as those with mental illness) or will prove expensive to treat (such as those with human immunodeficiency virus (HIV)–acquired immune deficiency syndrome (AIDS) and as a means of early identification of immigrants who would benefit from appropriate intervention (such as those with intestinal parasites, or who require immunization).

Table 9.6 Foreign-born population in the USA, poverty rates and health insurance coverage by region of birth, 1996

Region of birth	Population 1960 (millions)	Population 1997 (millions)	Poverty rate (%)	Health insurance Coverage (%)
Latin America	0.9	13.1	28.0	54.5
Asia	0.5	6.8	14.7	75.4
Europe	7.3	4.3	12.7	84.7
Other	1.1	1.5	17.1	66.5
US-born	–	–	12.9	86.3

Source: US Census Bureau (1999)

The third is that the circumstances of migration may themselves increase the risk of infectious disease. This is particularly so when there are movements of large numbers of internally displaced people and refugees in circumstances that are conducive to the spread of infectious disease. These include poor nutrition and sanitation, overcrowding, and lack of access to effective treatments. Failure to regulate and appropriately use antibiotics in such circumstances (a problem that is also very common in low-income countries and countries in which there is civil conflict or war) may also contribute to the emergence and spread of drug-resistant organisms.

These factors have contributed to the re-emergence of one of the leading infectious causes of death worldwide, tuberculosis (TB). It represents a spectacular failure of international disease control. The failure is not due to either lack of knowledge or lack of effective and inexpensive interventions – the disease is preventable and, in most cases, readily treatable. This failure, which is primarily due to the inequitable distribution of knowledge and resources, is a significant contributor to the rapid growth in drug-resistant TB in many parts of the world, in particular the countries of the former Soviet Union (Evans and Norris 2000; Farmer *et al.* 1999).

The importance of migration is illustrated by a study by Bakhshi *et al.* (1997) who report that the prevalence rates (per 100 000 population) of TB among ethnic groups in Birmingham, UK, were as follows: Caucasian – 9; Afro-Caribbean – 43; Asian – 150; and other – 59. They conclude that "from about the second decade of the next century, TB in the UK will almost be entirely a problem of ethnic minorities and that even if new infection was eliminated now in Asian people, cases due to reactivation would continue to occur until the third quarter of next century' (Bakhshi, Hawker & Ali, 1997).

More than 30 million people worldwide are infected with HIV. About 100 million people move voluntarily between and within countries each year, while a further 40 million are either internally displaced or refugees outside their own countries. Migrants are more vulnerable than local populations to acquiring HIV infection during migration (see Box 9.1) and spread the virus on return home (UNAIDS Joint United Nations Programme on HIV/AIDS and IOM 1998). A number of factors may link population mobility and increased risk of HIV infection:

♦ separation from family and social constraints, and a sense of anonymity, perhaps promoting greater sexual freedom and more high-risk sexual behaviour

♦ reduced availability of health and preventive services to immigrants and refugees

♦ living and working in conditions of poverty, powerlessness, social instability, social isolation, and loneliness.

Geographic mobility is one of the main facilitating conditions for HIV transmission in sub-Saharan Africa (Brockerhoff and Biddlecom 1999) with clear links between elevated HIV sero-prevalence and

♦ short duration of residency in a locality

♦ settlement or travel along major transportation routes

♦ immigrant status

♦ international travel to a region.

'Independent of marital and cohabitation status, social milieu, awareness of AIDS, and other crucial influences on sexual behaviour, male migrants between urban areas and female migrants within rural areas are much more likely than non-migrant counterparts to engage in sexual practices conducive to HIV infection' (Brockerhoff and Biddlecom 1999).

Despite the demonstrated relationship between the course of the HIV pandemic and human mobility, little specific policy development has focused on the relationship between population movement and HIV transmission (UNAIDS and IOM 1998).

Looking to the future, the combination of HIV and multi-resistant tuberculosis infection in some populations is likely to be catastrophic and will, almost certainly, raise public concerns about 'contagion' by migrants similar to those invoked by the appearance of cholera in Europe in the mid-nineteenth century.

Mental health

The prevalence of mental disorders among different immigrant groups is highly variable. Migration in itself is not associated with either increased or decreased risk for mental disorder (Klimidis *et al.* 1994). Among the groups most vulnerable to the development of mental health problems are refugees and asylum seekers. It is the specific circumstances of pre-migration experience, migration, and settlement that are important in influencing risk for mental disorder. Among these circumstances are the following.

- traumatic experiences or prolonged stress prior to or during migration
- being adolescent or elderly at the time of migration
- separation from family
- inability to speak the language of the host country
- prejudice and discrimination in the receiving society
- low socio-economic status and, even more critically, a drop in personal socio-economic status following migration
- non-recognition of occupational qualifications
- isolation from persons of a similar cultural background
- extent of acculturation.

A pattern of underutilization or overutilization of mental health services by particular groups may point to systematic inadequacies of a service system and raise important questions concerning needs for service, community attitudes towards and beliefs about mental illness and psychiatric treatment, barriers to service access, difficulties in diagnosis, and racism (Minas 2001).

Numerous studies have demonstrated differential service utilization by immigrant groups (Klimidis *et al.* 1999*a,b*; McDonald and Steel 1997). There are three broad factors that will influence the patterns of service use by different sections of the community (Klimidis *et al.* 2000). They are differences in prevalence of mental illness, different rates of entry into the service system, and different rates of exit from the service system. Reduced rates of voluntary entry into the service system may occur as a result of greater stigmatization of mental illness and psychiatric treatment; lack of knowledge of the availability of mental health services and of how to gain access to them; a preference for other forms of assistance (for example herbalist, priest); and failure of recognition of the presence of mental disorder at a primary care level. Increased rates of entry may occur as a result of misdiagnosis; lack of other more appropriate service options; and greater rates of compulsory admission and admission to secure units. Increased rates of exit from the service system may occur as a result of dissatisfaction with important elements of the service; services being seen as culturally insensitive; and increased stigma being associated with psychiatric treatment.

The most consistent pattern reported is one of under-utilization of mental health services by many ethnic communities in many different mental health service systems, although there is considerable variation by country of birth and, more particularly, by level of fluency in the language of the country concerned (Klimidis *et al.* 1999*a,b*; McDonald and Steel 1997).

There is relatively little information available on the quality of treatment outcome among cultural minority groups, although there are suggestions that outcome is generally poorer for immigrants (Minas *et al.* 1994).

A striking characteristic of the body of research into mental health of immigrants is the great variation in findings. The possible reasons for this lack of consistency include (Minas 2001)

(1) Wide variation in the demographic, cultural, and migration profiles of the groups being studied and the wide variation in national and regional mental health service systems.

(2) The many methodological difficulties that exist in cross-cultural mental health research (Minas 1996). These difficulties include lack of common definitions of the populations being studied, including problems with the concept of ethnicity; problems in sampling ethnic communities; lack of cross-culturally reliable and valid research instruments; problems associated with cross-cultural diagnosis; the lack of generally acceptable methods for studying culturally derived concepts of mental illness; and wide variations in clinical presentation across cultural groups and health systems.

Despite this variation, it is possible to conclude that many cultural minority groups in many different service systems experience difficulty in gaining access to culturally appropriate and effective mental health services (Minas 2001). A systematic effort is being made in a number of countries to ensure that mental health service systems develop the capacity to provide effective and culturally appropriate mental health services to populations that are characterized by cultural and linguistic diversity (Minas *et al.* 1993, 1995, 1996). Such efforts are either facilitated or constrained in different countries by national conceptions of citizenship and attitudes to diversity (Kirmayer and Minas 2000).

The role of health professionals

An intimate linkage has always existed between human mobility and disease. Migrants carry with them the specific disease burdens of the country from which they come. They are also exposed to new health risks during transit and in the country to which they migrate. They are also of course exposed to the health benefits of their adopted country. A basic issue is the crossing of biological and epidemiological boundaries as well as political and geographic boundaries, with differences in climate, pathogens, vectors, and lifestyles associated with good or poor health. The crossing of socio-cultural boundaries has significant implications for the migrant, for the receiving population, and for health professionals.

Immigrants and refugees generally have inequitable access to health services in countries of destination, and outcomes of health care services are often inferior to those for the host populations. There are data supporting these contentions in relation to immigrants and refugees in some countries, such as Australia and the UK. However, there is very little known about health status and access to health care services of immigrants and refugees in most parts of the world. There are many reasons for this lack of knowledge. In some cases it is simple indifference to their needs. In developing countries which have large numbers of immigrants and refugees the public health capacity that would be required to document the needs of immigrants and refugees and the capacity of health services to respond adequately to their needs is lacking. In a few countries there are cultural or even legal barriers to the research that is required. In Germany these have arisen in reaction to historical abuses of research on ethnicity. In France the conceptualization of the nation leads to a rejection of the idea of multi-culturalism (Kirmayer and Minas 2000). This is illustrated by that country's insistence on a reservation to its signature of the International Convention on Civil and Political Rights, in which it states that it does not recognize the existence of ethnic or linguistic minorities (Jack 1999). It is generally true that we know least about those sections of populations that have the greatest needs and where inequities are most marked.

Although the dynamics of emigration are complex, and intimately tied to broad political, social, and economic issues, it is clear that the key driver of migration, and the key determinant of population health differentials, is inequality. This inequality may be in a number of areas – economic, political, human rights, epidemiological, etc. Those aspects of globalization that result in increasing international inequalities will result in increased likelihood of migration, and in increased disparities in health status and access to health services. Those aspects of globalization that reduce international inequalities will reduce the pressure to migrate, and reduce the striking disparities in health status across nations.

There have been repeated phases of massive international migration over the centuries, with the most recent being during the decades following World War 2. Hirst and Thompson (1999) make the point that the period between 1815 and 1914 was much more open to migrants than the current period. The current era of 'globalization' is not associated with any freeing up of the internationalized market for labour. In fact, many countries (particularly the traditional migrant-receiving countries), have been making their criteria for accepting migrants and refugees more stringent.

The world's poor have fewer options for migration now than in much of history – constituting a substantial loss of freedom for the poor. However, the situation is the reverse for the wealthy and skilled. 'The 'club class' with managerial expertise, though relatively few in number in terms of the global population, are the most obvious manifestation of this inequity in long-term migratory opportunities' (Hirst and Thompson 1999).

Wars, civil disorder, environmental degradation, and natural disasters will continue to result in large numbers of refugees and internally displaced people, and to permanent and temporary labour migrants. While precisely where these events will occur is impossible to predict with accuracy, the fact of their continued occurrence is certain. An important international governance issue for nations and for international organizations will be how mobile labour is to be dealt with in a just and orderly manner, and how the world is to respond to the massive numbers of internally displaced people, asylum seekers, and refugees. An important part of this response is the extent to which attention is paid to the rights of labour migrants and refugees to adequate health protection and health care.

In the context of massive international migration and the profound economic, social, and cultural transformations that are occurring across the globe, the challenges that health professionals face are considerable. They have the opportunity to play an important role within the systems in which they work in a number of ways.

The first is in the area of health policy. Health professionals should work with national governments and local authorities to ensure that immigrants have equitable access to health services that are effective and appropriate to their needs. This is particularly important in relation to labour migrants, refugees, and asylum seekers, who are often excluded from existing health service arrangements as a matter of national health policy or through neglect.

The second is in the area of research. It is generally true that we know least about those populations, or sections of populations, whose needs are greatest (Global Forum for Health Research 1999). Health professionals should work to ensure that research is carried out that will enable health departments and health practitioners to understand health service needs of immigrants and refugees, plan appropriate services, and reduce existing health inequities.

The third area is education. Health professionals should be active in improving their own education in relation to working with immigrants and refugees who are from different cultural backgrounds (Minas 1999, 2000). They should also contribute to the development of community education and health promotion programmes that will ensure that immigrants and refugees are knowledgeable about protecting their own health, and are aware of, and can gain access to, the health services they require. Health professionals can play an important role in assisting immigrant communities to become active participants in the design, operation, and evaluation of health services.

A key contribution of health professionals in a globalizing world is a commitment to equity (Evans and Norris 2000; Whitehead 1992). Health is a primary good and a fundamental condition for the full exercise of rights and liberties. Health professionals are in a position to draw the attention of governments and society at large to the fact that basic institutions and social arrangements are inherently unjust if those institutions and arrangements themselves result in systematic disadvantage accruing to some social groups (Rawls 1997, 1993). They can contribute substantially to the reduction of such injustice.

Acknowledgement

This chapter is a revised version of an invited paper prepared for a meeting on equitable and efficient health sector strategies held at the Rockefeller Foundation Bellagio Study and Conference Centre, Italy, 3–7 July 2000. I am grateful to the convenors of the meeting, Professor Margaret Whitehead and Professor Göran Dahlgren, for inviting me to participate, and to the Rockefeller Foundation for making the meeting possible.

Box 9.1: Labour migration and HIV–AIDS

Incidence of HIV–AIDS is highest in economically less-developed countries.

Socio-political marginalization is associated with increased risk of HIV infection.

What are the factors among labour migrants that increase their risk of HIV infection?

(1) Labour migrants are among the poorest. They have limited access to information including preventive health information. In mots sending countries (for example Bangaldesh, Cambodia, India, Indonesia, Pakistan, Philippines, Sri Lanka, Vietnam) labour migrants receive little useful pre-departure information on HIV–AIDS and other STDs.

(2) At least half of labour migrants are women. Most women are employed as domestic workers and as workers in other low-skilled occupations, where they are at risk of abuse and sexual exploitation. Many of these women are subjected to violence, including sexual violence, during the pre-departure period and in the receiving country. For example, Indonesian migrant workers recruited by migration agents often from poor rural areas without a prior demand from prospective employers, are housed in overcrowded agency houses in very poor conditions.

(3) Undocumented migrants are at particular risk during the transit phase.

(4) A number of countries (for example Malaysia) have mandatory HIV testing and deportation rules for foreign workers. Their situation on return to the home country is unenviable.

(5) Foreign workers often have very limited access to health information and health care in the receiving country. Undocumented migrants often have no entitlement to health care and are reluctant to access health care for fear of discovery and deportation.

Box 9.1: **Labour migration and HIV–AIDS** (continued)

(6) Most countries receiving foreign temporary workers do not allow the worker's family to join them. This promotes sexual behaviour that is associated with increased risk of HIV infection.

(7) The employment of foreign workers is usually on the basis of bilateral agreements between sending and receiving countries. Sending countries are usually in a weak position to negotiate the rights of the foreign workers.

(8) The protection of the rights of foreign workers is a regional and international responsibility and requires multi-lateral agreements in relation to:

- labour protection
- mandatory HIV testing and deportation
- pre-departure programs that prepare workers to protect their health and their rights.

(9) Access to adequate health care in the receiving country.

Source Verghis 2000

References

Australian Institute of Health and Welfare (2000) *Australia's health 2000*, AIHW Cat No 19. Australia Government Publishing Service, Canberra.

Bakhshi, S. S., Hawker, J., and Ali, S. (1997) The epidemiology of tuberculosis by ethnic group in Birmingham and its implications for future trends in tuberculosis in the UK. *Ethnicity and Health*, **2**, 147–53.

Brockerhoff, M. and Biddlecom, A. E. (1999) Migration, sexual behaviour and the risk of HIV in Kenya. *International Migration Review*, **33**, 833–56.

Castles, S. (1999) International migration and the global agenda: reflections on the 1998 UN technical symposium. *International Migration Review*, **37**, 3–17.

Castles, S. and Miller, M. J. (1998) *The age of migration: international population movements in the modern world*. Guildford, New York.

Chin, C. B. N. (1997) Walls of silence and late twentieth century representations of the foreign female domestic worker: the case of Filipina and Indonesian Female servants in Malaysia. *International Migration Review*, **31**, 353–85.

Diatta, M. A. and Mbow, N. (1999) Releasing the development potential of return migration: the case of Senegal. *International Migration Review*, **37**, 243–64.

Editorial (1996) Organized crime moves into migrant trafficking. *Trafficking in Migrants Quarterly Bulletin (International Organization for Migration)*, **10**, 1–2.

Editorial (1997*a*) Prostitution in Asia increasingly involves trafficking. *Trafficking in Migrants Quarterly Bulletin (International organization for Migration)*, **11**, 1–2.

Editorial (1997*b*) Infectious disease and migration, Migration and Health Newsletter (International Organization for Migration), **1**, 1–3.

Editorial (1998) Migration medical screening: a move towards public health risk management. *Migration and Health Newsletter (International Organization for Migration)*, **2**, 1–3.

Evans, T. and Norris, A. (2000) Policy-oriented strategies for health equity. In *Efficient, equity-oriented strategies for health: international perspectives, focus on Vietnam*, ed. H. M. Pham, Y. Liu, I. H. Minas *et al.* Centre for International Mental Health, Melbourne.

Farmer, P. (1996) Social inequalitieis and emerging infectious diseases. *Emerging Infectious Diseases*, **2**, 259–68.

Farmer, P. E., Reichman, L. B., and Iseman, M. D. (1999) *The global impact of drug resistant tuberculosis.* Harvard Medical School/Open Society Institute, Boston.

Freeman, G. P. (1995) Modes of immigration politics in liberal democratic states. *International Migration Review*, **29**, 881–902.

Global Forum for Health Research (1999) The 10/90 report on health research. WHO, Geneva.

Green, J. R. (1992) *A short history of the English people.* The Folio society, London.

Hirst, P. and Thompson, G. (1996) *Globalization in question: the international economy and the possibilities of governance.* Polity Press, Cambridge.

Hirst, P. and Thompson, G. (1999) *Globalization in question*, 2nd edn. Polity Press, Cambridge.

Huntington, S. P. (1996) *The clash of civilizations and the remaking of world order.* Simon & Schuster, New York.

Jack, A. (1999) *The french exception.* Profile Books, London.

Keely, C. B. (1996) How nation-states create and respond to refugee flows. *International Migration Review*, **30**, 1046–66.

Kirmayer, L. J. and Minas, I. H. (2000) The future of cultural psychiatry: an international perspective. *Canadian Journal of Psychiatry*, **45**, 438–46.

Klimidis, S., Stuart, G., Minas, I. H. *et al.* (1994) Immigrant status and gender effects on psychopathology and self-concept in adolescents: a test of the migration-morbidity hypothesis. *Comprehensive Psychiatry*, **35**, 393–404.

Klimidis, S., Lewis, J., Miletic, T. *et al.* (1999*a*) Mental health service use by ethnic communities in Victoria: Part I, descriptive report. http://www.ccsh.unimelb.edu.au/vtpu/mhsu/leader.pdf. Victorial Transcultural Psychiatry Unit, Melbourne.

Klimidis, S., Lewis, J., Miletic, T. *et al.* (1999*b*) Mental health service use by ethnic communities in Victoria: Part II, statistical tables. http://www.ccsh.unimelb.edu.au.vtpu/mhsu/leader.pdf. Victorial Transcultural Psychiatry Unit, Melbourne.

Klimidis, S., McKenzie, D. P., Lewis, J. *et al.* (2000) Continuity of contact with psychiatric services: immigrant and Australian-born patients. *Social Psychiatry and Psychiatric Epidemiology*, **35**, 554–563.

Kraut, A. (1994) Historial aspects of refugee and immigration movements. In *Amidst peril and pain: the mental health and wel-being of the world's refugees*, ed. A. J. Marsella, T. Bornemann, S. Ekblad *et al.* American Psychological Association, Washington DC.

Marsella, A. J. (1994) Ethnocultural diversity and international refugees: challenge for the global community. In *Amidst peril and pain: the mental health and wel-being of the world's refugees*, ed. A. J. Marsella, T. Bornemann, S. Ekblad *et al.* American Psychological Association, Washington DC.

McBride, M. J. (1999) Migrants and asylum seekers: policy responses in the United States to immigrants and refugees from Central America and the Caribbean. *International Migration*, **37**, 289–314.

McDonald, R. and Steel, Z. (1997) *Immigrants and mental health: an epidemiological analysis.* Transcultural Mental Health Centre, Sydney.

Minas, I. H. (1996) Transcultural psychiatry. *Current Opinion in Psychiatry,* **9**, 144–8.

Minas, I. H. (1999) Cross-cultural training for health professionals. In *Cultural dimensions: approaches to diversity training in Australia,* ed. Human Rights and Equal Opportunity Commissioner. Human Rights and Equal Opportunity Commission, Sydney

Minas, I. H. (2000) Culture and psychiatric education. *Australasian Psychiatry,* **8**, 204–6.

Minas, I. H. (2001) Service responses to cultural diversity. In *Textbook of community psychiatry,* ed. G. Thornicroft and G. Szmukler, pp. 193–206. Oxford University Press, Oxford.

Minas, I. H., Silove, D., and Kunst, J. P. (1993) Mental health for multicultural Australia: a national strategy. Report of a consultancy to the Commonwealth Department of Human Services and Health. Victorial Transcultural Psychiatry Unit, Melbourne.

Minas, I. H., Stuart, G. W., and Klimidis, S. (1994) Language, culture and psychiatric services: a survey of Victorian clinical staff. *Australian and New Zealand Journal of Psychiatry,* **28**, 250–8.

Minas, I. H., Ziguras, S., Klimidis, S. *et al.* (1995) *Extending the framework: a proposal for a statewide bilingual clinical support and development program.* Victorian Transcultural Psychiatry Unit, Melbourne.

Minas, I. H., Lambert, T. J. R., Kostov, S. *et al.* (1996) *Mental health service for NESB immigrants: transforming policy into practice.* Austalian Government Publishing Service, Canberra.

Morse, S. (1995) Factors in the emergence of infectious diseases. *Emerging Infectious Disease,* **1**, 7–15.

Rawls, J. (1971) *A theory of justice.* Harvard University Press, Cambridge.

Rawls, J. (1993) *Political liberalism.* Columbia University Press, New York.

Roberts, K. D. (1997) China's "tidal wave" of migrant labour: what can we learn from Mexican undocumented migration to the United States? *International Migration Review,* **31**, 249–93.

Salt, J. and Stein, J. (1997) Migration as a business: the case of trafficking. *International Migration Review,* **35**, 467–91.

Segal, A. (1993) *Atlas of international migration.* Hans Zell, London.

Taran, P. (1999) Seven causes of migration in the age of globalisation. International migration policy and law course for Asia Pacifique. November 1999, Bangkok, Thailand.

Tomas, P. S. (1999) Enhancing the capabilities of emigration countries to protect men and women destined for low-skilled employment: the case of the Philippines. *International Migration Review,* **37**, 319–51.

UNAIDS and IOM (1998) Migration and AIDS. *International Migration,* **36**, 445–66.

US Census Bureau (1999) Current population reports. Series P23–195, profile of the foreign-born population in the United States, 1997. US Government Printing Office, Washington DC.

US Committee for Refugees (1999) World refugee survey 1999. Immigration and Refugee Services of America, Washington.

Verghis, S. (2000) Promoting and protecting human rights to reduce HIB vulnerability of migrant workers, http://www.gn.apc.org/caramasia/sharuna_paper.htm.

Whitehead, M. (1992) Concepts and principles of equity and health. *International Journal of Health Services,* **22,** 429–45.

World Bank (1996) *World development report 1996: from plan to market.* Oxford University Press, New York.

Zlotnik, H. (1999) Trends of international migration since 1965: what existing data reveal. *International Migration,* **37,** 21–59.

Chapter 10

International co-operation for reproductive health: too much ideology?

Louisiana Lush and Oona Campbell

Introduction

The burden of reproductive ill health is one of the world's most serious health problems. Each year around 600 000 women die and many more encounter serious problems in childbirth (World Health Organization (WHO) 1996; AbouZahr 1998). In 1995 there were 330 million new sexually transmitted infections (STIs) (WHO/Global Programme on AIDS 1995), and in 1999 an estimated 5.6 million new cases of human immunodeficiency virus (HIV) (UNAIDS 1999). Furthermore 120 million women had unwanted pregnancies in 1990 and there were 20 million unsafe abortions (Ashford 1995). The vast majority of these problems occurred in low-income countries, where poverty increases sickness and reduces access to care. Reproductive health problems are also increasingly seen within a context of gender-based economic, political, and cultural discrimination and neglect of women's rights to equal status and equitable access to services. Gender discrimination often interacts with poverty, such that women in low-income countries face many obstacles to personal, social, and financial security. These disadvantages increase women's vulnerability to ill health and reduce their ability to protect themselves or get help for their problems. Reproductive health was defined at the International Conference on Population and Development (ICPD) as (United Nations (UN) 1995a)

> a state of complete physical, mental and social well-being and not merely the absence of diseases or infirmity, in all matters relating to the reproductive system and to its functions and processes. [It] therefore implies that people are able to have a satisfying and safe sex life and that they have the capability to reproduce and the freedom to decide if, when and how often to do so

This health definition was conceptualized within a social, economic, and political context, founded on the basic rights of women and men to safe and voluntary sex and childbearing, a concept which was further endorsed by the Fourth International Women's Conference in Beijing in 1995 (UN 1995b).

Since the late 1980s there has been increased international recognition of and co-operation over reproductive health problems, led by such agencies as the WHO and the World Bank and helped by the knowledge that many problems are relatively cheap and easy to solve. For example, three of the top five most cost-effective interventions for reducing disease burden among adults address preventing unwanted pregnancy, treating STIs and preventing maternal mortality (World Bank 1993). In 1994 these concerns received global attention at the ICPD in Cairo, organized by the UN Population Fund (UNFPA) and attended by government delegations from 180 countries as well as some 1200 non-governmental organizations (NGOs).

In this chapter we address the process by which reproductive health came to such international prominence in the early 1990s through a focus on the international actors involved and the process of negotiation between them. We then examine two high priority areas of reproductive health care in detail: efforts to reduce maternal mortality and efforts to integrate HIV/STI and family planning services. In so doing, we aim to illustrate two features of international co-operation for health: first, how the process of global agenda setting was driven by a relatively small set of international actors with particular ideologies; and second, how, despite relatively simple and cheap technologies being available, this process of agenda setting in fact limited the effectiveness with which appropriate interventions were implemented.

Technical definitions of problems and solutions

Unwanted pregnancy

Unwanted pregnancy and associated unmet need for family planning have long been a major concern internationally due to their associations with fertility levels and population growth. Measured regularly through the international Demographic and Health Surveys, between 11 and 40 per cent of women were defined as having an unmet need for family planning in 1985–89 (Westoff and Ochoa 1991). These figures included women who stated either that they would rather have delayed the pregnancy in question or not had it at all. Such pregnancies are deemed to have been preventable had better quality and more accessible family planning services been available. In general, women of higher education or income levels or those living in urban areas had a greater demand for birth control.

In the 1970s and 1980s, such ideas guided the development of a wide range of innovative approaches to family planning service delivery around the world. The core of a family-planning programme remains clinic-based, with services sometimes provided by a specialist nurse/midwife but usually through general primary health care (PHC) services. However, other approaches have also proved successful in increasing access to care for a wide sector of the population, including extending the range of methods available at specialized clinics to include surgical, clinical, and non-clinical methods; community-based service delivery through voluntary but trained providers; and social marketing of hormonal contraceptives and condoms through private shops and pharmacies at subsidized prices (Ross *et al.* 1992). Through these many different approaches, large numbers of women around the world have gained access to family planning even where other health care is unavailable.

Services were traditionally guided by concerns with population growth and associated with targets for 'a couple of years of protection' or 'numbers of new acceptors'

(Ross *et al.* 1992). In recent years this approach has been heavily criticized as leading to potentially or actually coercive measures, based on evidence from such countries as India, China, and Indonesia (Bose 1989; Hesketh and Zhu 1997). In response, family-planning programmes shifted somewhat away from inundation approaches and towards a more client-oriented focus, based on major developments in understanding with provision of better quality care (Jain *et al.* 1992).

Maternal mortality

Nearly all the 585 000 women who die each year of maternal causes are from developing countries (WHO 1996). Three-quarters die from five main 'direct' obstetrical complications: haemorrhage, sepsis, hypertensive diseases of pregnancy, obstructed labour, and unsafe abortion (AbouZahr 1998). Maternal deaths affect hundreds of thousands of families and communities; several million children are left motherless each year, and an estimated one million young children die soon after the deaths of their mothers. Adding maternal morbidity to mortality, the 1993 World Bank global burden of disease exercise estimated that 18 per cent of the disease burden of women aged 15–49 was due to maternal causes, making maternal health problems the leading cause of ill health in this age group (World Bank 1993).

The scope to reduce the five main causes of maternal death with preventive measures is limited. Access to contraception and safe abortion services would reduce deaths among unwanted pregnancies in general and play a big role in preventing deaths from induced abortion. However, neither service is relevant to women who actually want to give birth. Antenatal care is the traditional preventive arm of maternal health services. By the early 1990s however, many argued that the antenatal 'high-risk screening' approach promoted in the 1970s and 1980s (Backett *et al.* 1984) was ineffective (Maine 1991). Many other antenatal activities have never been shown to be effective (for example, promotion of healthy eating); others are effective but target either the neonate or maternal morbidity but not mortality (for example, tetanus toxoid immunization or STI screening and treatment). This limits effective activities likely to reduce maternal mortality to a few, such as detection and treatment of pre-eclampsia before it becomes severe and presumptive treatment of all women with sulphadoxine–pyrimethamine to prevent severe anaemia due to malaria (Rooney 1992; Shulman *et al.* 1999). In terms of delivery services, aseptic techniques can reduce the risk of infection, the partograph appears to improve management of labour, and leads to better outcomes with respect to obstructed labour, and oxytocic drugs given in the third stage of delivery reduce post-partum haemorrhage. The last two in particular rely on the presence of skilled personnel.

Preventing the bulk of maternal deaths thus requires curative care, that is, using clinical services to treat conditions as they arise to prevent them from leading to death (WHO 1991). Fortunately, starting in the mid–1930s, medical technologies were developed to deal effectively with these complications (Loudon 1992). In the west, childbirth was professionalized and increasingly institutionalized; maternal mortality declined dramatically and ceased to be a major public health concern (Loudon 1992). In other countries, national policies seem to have depended to a great extent on the prevailing political systems and the allegiances held by governments in the Cold War

(Zapata and Godue 1997). In general, socialist countries prioritized health care as a human right and made maternal health facilities widely available, including community programmes in the rural areas and abortion services (Rosenfield and Maine 1985). In the western-oriented developing countries maternal health and access to health-care in general was less of a priority to policy makers and donors.

During the 1980s the promotion of minimally trained multi-purpose workers at the community level, including traditional and volunteer health cadres that did not need government salaries, was a development in harmony with the thrusts of both PHC and cost containment. As part of this trend in the 1970s and 1980s, training of traditional birth attendants (TBAs) was seen as a solution (Belsey 1985; WHO 1974), but came to be discredited by the 1990s. In the poorest countries, coverage of professional delivery care services remained severely restricted, irrespective of ideology; levels of maternal mortality remained very high.

In 1987, the Safe Motherhood Conference in Nairobi drew attention to the persisting tragedy of maternal death in developing countries and set itself a target to halve maternal deaths by the year 2000 (Mahler 1987). The challenge for developing countries is to organize health services that deliver relevant preventive and curative interventions, particularly around the time of labour and delivery when most deaths occur. To be successful, safe-motherhood programmes must decrease the gap between women and services so that both respond rapidly and appropriately to the obstetrical complications which cause death.

HIV/AIDS and other sexually transmitted infections

By the end of 1997, the HIV virus had infected a cumulative total of more than 47 million people globally, 33 million of whom were still alive (UNAIDS 1998a). Of these, most were under 30 years old and 10 per cent of new infections in 1997 were among children under 15, mostly infected from their mothers. The consequences of HIV infection are grave: according to the WHO, HIV/acquired immune deficiency syndrome (AIDS) is the fourth biggest cause of death worldwide and in Africa it is now the leading single cause of death, at 19 per cent of all deaths (WHO 1999). The impact on the societies and economies where the disease is highly prevalent has been huge: like maternal mortality but unlike other causes of death, which strike mainly the elderly and the very young, HIV/AIDS kills the most economically productive people, aged 25–40 years. The result is a host of macro- and micro-level, household and business, and individual and community effects which will dramatically slow development in countries which have severe epidemics (Ainsworth and Over 1994; Bloom and Godwin 1997; International Labour Organisation 1995; Over 1998).

In low-income countries, opportunities for treating HIV/AIDS or associated opportunistic infections have been limited by the high cost of effective drugs. Efforts to control the disease have therefore emphasized primary prevention, including condom promotion, health and sex education, and raising awareness about risks associated with certain patterns of sexual behaviour (De Cock et al. 1994; Adler et al. 1998;). However, despite over a decade of efforts, by the mid–1990s few successes had been documented, largely due to the extreme political and cultural difficulties of addressing highly sensitive and personal areas of behaviour (Caldwell et al. 1992).

In the early 1990s, therefore, the emphasis of HIV prevention efforts shifted from behaviour change education to controlling other STIs. While STIs were not a new problem themselves, they received increased attention as evidence emerged on their role in facilitating HIV infection (Cohen 1998). The 1993 World Development Report stated that STIs, excluding HIV, accounted for nine per cent of the total burden of disease among adult women, second only to maternal factors, and nearly two per cent of the burden of disease among men (World Bank 1993). Sexually transmitted infections can lead to chronic pain, infertility, pelvic inflammatory disease, abortion, neo-natal infection, and death. Women are more likely to suffer from long-term adverse consequences of these infections than men, because their reproductive systems are more vulnerable and the diseases are less likely to show symptoms and be treated (Gerbase *et al.* 1998; Holmes and Ryan 1999).

Infection with an STI, either ulcerative or non-ulcerative, among both men and women, is now known to be strongly associated with a greatly increased risk of HIV transmission (Wasserheit 1992; Cohen 1998). The link with HIV has been found for a large number of STIs, including gonorrhoea, chlamydia, genital ulcers, and trichomoniasis, although much less is known about quantifying this risk or the extent to which asymptomatic STIs also contribute to increased HIV risk (Grosskurth 1999). In 1995, the results of a community-based, randomized, controlled trial in Mwanza district, Tanzania showed that HIV incidence in the intervention areas could be reduced to 38 per cent below that in control areas as a result of a range of new activities: syndromic management of presenting STIs; community awareness raising of services; condom promotion; partner tracing; and enhanced supervision of medical staff (Grosskurth *et al.* 1995; Hayes *et al.* 1995). The intervention was also found to be highly cost effective, at US$10 per disability-adjusted life year (DALY) (Gilson *et al.* 1997). The DALY is defined by the World Bank (1993) as

> a unit used for measuring both the global burden of disease and the effectiveness of health interventions, as indicated by reductions in the disease burden. It is calculated as the present value of the future years of disability-free life that are lost as the result of the premature deaths or cases of disability occurring in a particular year

Relative to other primary level services, such as child immunization, which cost between US$12–17 per DALY, this intervention is considered to be highly cost-effective. The outcome of this study was a renewed interest in STIs in low-income countries and the extent to which they were contributing to the rapid spread of HIV. However, most recent research shows that this intervention is less effective for women: first, because few STIs in women have any symptoms at all so they do not present for treatment (Behets *et al.* 1995; Ryan *et al.* 1998); and second, symptoms which do appear are not easily attributed to particular infectious agents for treatment (Hawkes *et al.* 1999).

International policy actors in reproductive health

While the scientific rationale for each of these different reproductive health interventions was relatively clear, moving from research evidence to international co-operation and policy development was a complex process, involving a wide range of actors with different interests and influence. In this section, we follow the agendas of the main actors from the mid–1960s until the mid–1990s.

Family planning actors

During the 1960s and early 1970s, neither maternal health nor STIs were considered serious health problems internationally, and HIV was unrecognized. Family-planning policy, meanwhile, was driven by a macro-economic agenda of concern over the impact of rapid population growth on developing economies. This concern led to the development of vertically funded and managed family-planning programmes, heavily prioritized by international donors, in particular, the United States Agency for International Development (USAID) (Finkle and McIntosh 1994). UNFPA was founded in 1969, with the Filipino Raphael Salas as its first Executive Director, and mandated to fund population activities through other UN agencies' national offices. Around this time, a number of international family-planning NGOs were also established, including the Population Council, and large US-based foundations, such as Rockefeller and Ford, began to take a significant interest in population issues (Finkle and McIntosh 1994).

Family-planning policy, however, was rarely without controversy and both the 1974 and 1984 population conferences, in Bucharest and Mexico City respectively, saw rifts between major groups of actors with different agendas on the table. At Bucharest, the main debate was between developing countries, led by the recently formed New International Economic Order (NIEO), and the US government, heavily influenced by environmentalists' concerns over a global population explosion. The NIEO, by contrast, demanded less attention to purely population issues and more assistance for general development, which they saw as leading inevitably to slower population growth: 'development is the best contraceptive' (Lee and Walt 1995). The period after Bucharest saw an expansion of population activities around the world, including the development of UNFPA into an agency with its own national offices and representatives, thus freeing it from dependence on other UN agencies with competing priorities (Finkle and McIntosh 1994). Actors involved in population and health agendas intersected in a variety of ways and each sought to use the other's platform. The health benefits of family planning were highlighted to legitimize contraception (WHO 1974), while advocates of child health sought to garner the resources available for population activities by arguing that lower child mortality would lead to lower fertility (Taylor *et al.* 1976).

At national level, the greatest successes for family-planning policies in this period were seen among south and south-east Asian governments, with strong family-planning programmes being established in many countries and the onset of fertility declines in many populations around the region (Finkle and McIntosh 1994). Governments in sub-Saharan Africa, by contrast, undertook little programme development and family planning remained steadfastly unpopular among the general population. Similarly, strong religious opposition heavily influenced Latin American governments and so they established NGOs to provide services to increasingly well-educated populations with modern demands for birth control.

By the 1984 Mexico City population conference, the agenda was radically different although no less fraught with difficulty: developing countries had lost much of their economic optimism of the 1960s and 1970s and were desperate for assistance of any kind; many more countries had established family-planning programmes although resource constraints hindered their activities. The USA, meanwhile, under the new-right Reagan administration, was more responsive to the religious, especially Catholic, lobby and was reducing its commitments to international family-planning programmes (McIntosh and Finkle 1995). At the same time, it strengthened its support for child survival programmes (Reich 1995). In the period following the Mexico City conference, the international family-planning policy community changed further with the entrance of new actors, such as the World Bank, and the growth of resistance to the coercive approaches of population control among international women's organizations. Thus while population policy was still driven largely by an economic rationale, and attracted the large funds available from the World Bank on this basis, it also developed more sophisticated ways of recruiting clients through improving the quality and accessibility of its services (Jain *et al.* 1992).

Maternal health actors

International co-operation in maternal health started in the mid–1960s, when western donor countries and international agencies first started to fund maternal and child health (MCH) programmes of national Ministries of Health. However, throughout the 1970s, those involved in maternal health were influenced by the family-planning movement. The WHO, one of the earliest actors to write on the issue of maternal health (Vaughan 1987), clearly adopted and prioritized a family planning strategy in one of its first documents on maternal health (WHO 1974). For other actors too, such as the UN Children's Fund (UNICEF) and USAID, the focus and funding of MCH was actually geared to child health and family planning (Rosenfield and Maine 1985).

The WHO remained a key actor in the late 1970s and early 1980s as a new health care ideology was promoted for developing countries. This involved switching towards PHC and the proposal of 'Health for All by the Year 2000'. The WHO's approach to maternal health in the mid–1980s advises training TBAs as one of the most cost-effective strategies to reduce maternal mortality and morbidity (Belsey 1985). Traditional birth attendant training programmes also drew considerable support and funds from UNICEF, UNFPA, and USAID, among others, especially since the latter two agencies had a further interest in using TBAs as family-planning workers.

During the same period, the international women's health movement, which had emerged in the 1970s in the industrialized west, started to lead global campaigns for women's rights and to expand the interest in women's health beyond family planning. Government donor agencies, such as the Swedish Agency for Research Co-operation with Developing Countries (SAREC), foundations, and NGOs also supported research and activities in women's health (for example, see Bergstrom *et al.* 1992; World Federation of Public Health Associations 1986). The Women in Development programme within USAID also supported research-based activities on women's health issues through an NGO, the International Centre for Research on Women (ICRW). The women's movement also brought the issue of maternal health success-fully to the attention of major international institutions like the WHO and the World Bank. They made a public outcry about the high levels of maternal mortality in the developing world at the Mexico City Population Conference of 1984 and the World Conference to Review and Appraise the Achievements of the UN Decade for Women in Nairobi in 1985. The World Bank itself was also to play a key role: in the 1980s they attempted to counterbalance the child survival work that had been led by USAID, UNICEF and, to a lesser extent, the WHO and redress the balance in favour of adult health (Reich 1993).

Finally, in 1985, two academics from Columbia University, Rosenfield and Maine (1985) wrote a highly influential paper that served as a watershed to galvanize interest and to put the issue of maternal mortality on the international health policy agenda. They argued that MCH programmes focused almost exclusively on child health, assuming that 'whatever is good for the child is good for the mother' (Rosenfield and Maine 1985), and called on obstetricians and the World Bank to take the lead in maternal health policy. The first international conference devoted to maternal mor-tality (Safe Motherhood Conference, Nairobi, Kenya, 10–13 February 1987) was spon-sored by the World Bank, the WHO and UNFPA and led to the launch of the Safe Motherhood Initiative (SMI).

International agencies involved in the SMI coalition included five UN agencies (the WHO, the UN Development Programme (UNDP), the World Bank, UNFPA, and UNICEF) and two NGOs (the Population Council and International Planned Parenthood Federation). Family Care International, another NGO, also came to be involved in organizing the first national conferences on safe motherhood. The United States Agency for International Development was not a SMI coalition member but was influential through its 'MotherCare' demonstration projects and research sup-port. Other, mainly research, activities were also launched in response. These include the Columbia University Prevention of Maternal Mortality Network in West Africa, funded initially by the Carnegie Foundation (Lucas 1997); the London School of Hygiene and Tropical Medicine Methods for Measuring Maternal Health Programme, supported by the Ford Foundation and the UK Overseas Development Administration (now Department for International Development (DFID)) (Graham and Campbell 1990); and the Uppsala University International Maternal Health Care Training Programme, supported by the Swedish Agency for International, Technical and Economic Co-operation (BITS) (Bergstrom et al. 1993).

HIV actors

In the late 1980s, the HIV epidemic was recognized in low-income countries, especial-ly in sub-Saharan Africa. Early policy efforts were led by the Global Programme on AIDS (GPA), established in 1987 as a specialized programme within the WHO (Lee and Zwi 1996). The policy of GPA emphasized bio-medical approaches to disease control such as the prevention of high-risk behaviour and screening of blood dona-tions. Programmes were established in many countries around the world, again fund-ed and managed vertically, outside mainstream Ministry of Health systems. With a few exceptions, notably Thailand and Uganda, national government commitments to HIV/AIDS control were extremely weak, partly because of high levels of stigma and shame associated with the disease, at both individual and cultural levels (Caldwell *et al.* 1992). Early failures, therefore, led to a backlash to bio-medical approaches, which were seen as unhelpful in their focus on stigmatized, high-risk activities and subsequent blaming of infected individuals. In addition, the spread of HIV beyond traditional core groups necessitated a broader scope of prevention activities. The GPA was closed and UNAIDS established in its place in 1996 as a joint UN programme between many different UN agencies with a mandate to work with national governments to develop effective prevention activities (Lee and Zwi 1996).

The link between traditional STIs and HIV was established in the late 1980s and fed into efforts to establish new ways to address the HIV epidemic in the general population through existing health services (USAID 1995). By the mid–1990s, USAID had become much more heavily involved in HIV/AIDS funding and was the largest single donor to international HIV/AIDS control efforts (Delay 1998). Throughout, there were relatively few powerful NGOs active in HIV/AIDS or STI policy and the agenda was dominated by the UN, the WHO or other technical 'experts'. Only very recently, with the release of catastrophic epidemic data by UNAIDS (UNAIDS 1998*b*) has an international non-government alliance been established to develop innovative and cheap ways of preventing and treating HIV.

Ideological paradigms

Developments in family planning, maternal health, and integrated HIV/STI policies have all been guided by particular ideological paradigms. Beyond the obvious role played by economic rationales, the most prominent of these have been, first, the need to prioritize interventions which are appropriate for delivery at basic PHC facilities and, second, the desire to address health problems through improving the status of women. The various international policy actors involved have adopted these ideologies to varying degrees. To some extent this has been based on political expediency and presentation rather than technical or scientific evidence, a process which has led to problems with implementing effective health programmes at national level.

Primary health care

Since its origin in the 1960s and 1970s, PHC has been guided by five principles: equitable distribution, community involvement, focus on prevention, appropriate technology, and a multi-sectoral approach (Walt and Vaughan 1982). It was grounded in a broad theory of development that rejected economic modernization as the only means to human well-being and placed good health firmly at the centre of an economic growth–equity–productivity nexus. Furthermore, in the Alma Ata Declaration of 1978, the international public health community committed to comprehensive PHC as part of a broader political and economic development agenda (WHO 1978). For family planning, the PHC approach worked well, since services are generally clinically simple and cheap to provide widely. By contrast, for maternal health, implementing PHC translated into a limited set of activities, none of which were particularly effective. Similarly, in the 1970s, efforts to control STIs through vertical, specialist services were more effective then subsequent PHC-based services (Mayaud 2000).

During the 1980s, however, in an increasingly neo-liberal and resource-constrained global climate, these ideals ceded to selective care, based on what were perceived to be cheap service packages. This shift also reflected the growth in influence and financial commitment of richer and more economically motivated international actors, such as the World Bank (Walt 1998). The failures of PHC therefore came under intense scrutiny, especially the unrealistic nature of the original objectives, given levels of public sector expenditure, and the difficulties of ensuring equitable resource allocation (Chen 1986; Rifkin and Walt 1986; McPake *et al.* 1993; Collins and Green 1994; Kalumba 1997).

More recently, major reforms were initiated in many low-income countries to try to increase efficiency in health service financing, expand access to primary level services and improve quality of care (Berman 1995; Janovsky 1996). As part of this effort, international donors emphasized basic packages of care that were considered to be cheap and cost effective and should therefore be available to all. The most heavily promoted of these packages included services that primarily target women and their children, namely maternal health, immunization, family planning, and treatment and prevention of STIs (World Bank 1993). In ideal conditions, these packages were to be delivered through strengthened PHC systems, centred on decentralized district administrations that would have enhanced autonomy and responsibility, reflecting international concern to improve governance and efficiency simultaneously. In reality, however, many reforms have been driven more by the need to cut costs and increase efficiency than to improve quality of care or local accountability. This has taken place in an environment of declining funds for health care among both low-income country governments and donors.

Women's status

Women's status in low-income countries and its relationship with poor health outcomes has long been a cause for concern among western women's groups and increasingly among low-income country women's groups themselves. Associations between women's education, autonomy, and financial independence on the one hand and health problems, such as nutritional status, infant and child mortality, fertility, and access to health care, on the other hand, have long been described (Kabeer 1994). There is also a well-documented interaction between poverty and gender, by virtue of which poor women often live in extremely vulnerable situations with little access to education or income with which to protect themselves from impending disaster (Folbre 1983; Boserup 1989; Oppenheim Mason 1993).

Unlike with PHC, however, there is little international consensus over how to define or operationalize women's rights to greater autonomy and equality in the many different settings around the world. Considerable debate remains over what the goal is and what should be the means of achieving it (van Stavaren 1994; Basu 1997). Many feminists in low-income countries challenge western ideas, grounded in philosophies of individual freedom, as culturally insensitive in societies where family and community values remain important structural determinants of an individual's choices or behaviour (Oppenheim Mason 1993). Furthermore, they assert, by destroying many of these social structures, many economic development policies in fact contributed to the increased vulnerability of women (Agarwal 1994).

Nevertheless, during the 1980s, improving gender equality and women's rights became a central tenet of women's health activists' argument (Lane 1994), some going as far as to say that only by improving women's status could meaningful improvements in reproductive health be achieved, to the dismay of traditional population controllers (Cleland 1996). While the status of the girl child received early attention from international policy makers, problems that afflict women in reproductive age groups, including the previously neglected categories of adolescents and unmarried women only became more prominent recently. Thus, the literature has highlighted, for example, the lack of power women have over the risky sexual behaviour of their partners (De Cock *et al.* 1994). Within the international women's movement, there was a long and intense feminist debate over whether contraception is a liberating phenomenon or an attempt by powerful sectors of society to control fertility among disadvantaged groups (for a review of early debates, see Folbre 1992).

Politics of decisions in the lead-up to the International Conference on Population and Development

Interactions between the wide range of actors involved in policy making and these two international ideological debates contributed to the process by which the agenda at the ICPD emerged as a radical new consensus. To understand the process of establishing such a consensus, the actors involved and their networks of communication and political interests will now be examined. The two networks that were particularly important in determining this agenda were the international women's movement and the international donor community, that is, the aid agencies representing western governments (McIntosh and Finkle 1995). (The term 'international women's movement' is used to denote the many women's rights advocacy groups and points of view that were most influential in determining the reproductive health agenda; at the same time, it must be recognized that these were a diverse set of actors and organizations with different interests and positions. It is their coming together during the pre-ICPD period that is of interest here.) In the period leading up to the ICPD, there was a strong effort by the international women's movement to publicize their agenda of shifting the rationale of family-planning programmes from population control to improving women's health. Organizations such as the International Women's Health Coalition (IWHC) and Family Care International and Development Alternatives for Women (DAWN) were established during this period and were significant in mobilizing support for the new agenda through a series of international meetings. Through the IWHC and other similar bodies, links with NGOs in low-income countries were strengthened in order to foster support for the new agenda and to present it as a global goal rather than one of rich countries alone (Germain and Kyte 1995). These networks were in theory facilitating global participation in determining the agenda; in reality, drafts of the document were prepared in New York and reflected priorities set by actors there (Petchesky 1995). Furthermore, their efforts at advocacy and drawing attention to the issues facing women in poor countries were more successful than the search for cheap, simple, and effective interventions to the major health problems.

In 1992, a more receptive political environment in the USA was presented by the replacement of the Reagan administration by Clinton. In this context, women's activists were able to raise attention to the low status of women and its relationship with both poverty and demographic outcomes and thereby also contribute to the changing emphasis of family-planning programmes (Germain 1987; Hartmann 1987; Garcia-Moreno and Claro 1994). Similarly, in a shifting international political economy, low-income country women's groups attacked neo-liberal development models as having increased poverty and hardship for women (Sen *et al.* 1994). These activities culminated in the publication in 1993 of the Women's Declaration on Population Policies, just before the second official Prepcom for the ICPD ('Prepcom' became the term used for a series of three formal preparatory committees which were held in the four years prior to the ICPD at regional and international level; they aimed to forge consensus and gain representation from a wide range of actors around the world at an early stage of development and drafting of the Programme of Action.). This changing agenda led to the incorporation of previously separate areas of health into the definition of reproductive health, including maternal health and HIV/STIs. Those involved in maternal health policy were mainly concerned with ensuring that maternal health was part of this agenda for advocacy purposes, in the hope of attracting greater financial resources.

Pressure and advocacy continued up to the conference and the wide recognition of the reproductive health agenda was the direct result of these efforts (McIntosh and Finkle 1995). As a result, senior decision makers in international donors were persuaded that the new approach was feasible and appropriate to the time: for example, there were an unprecedented 35 UN-sponsored preparatory meetings and consultations held all over the world in the years before the conference (see issues of *Population and Development Review*, 1992–1993). At these regional and national meetings, government and NGO representatives met together to determine priorities for the conference and to discuss and amend early drafts of the Programme of Action. By the time of the conference, only a few controversial issues remained to be resolved, including statements on abortion, sexual rights, and adolescent reproductive health. Despite the relatively low involvement of either maternal health or HIV/STI policy communities in defining the reproductive health agenda, women's groups saw both sets of services as core elements of a comprehensive reproductive health care package.

Western governments, meanwhile, initially took a more conservative stance and rejected women's groups' efforts to shift attention from family planning to a broader package of care (McIntosh and Finkle 1995). The USA, which had long been the most important funder of population activities, was however, in a position to take on a new role, with the decline of the new right and the arrival of the Clinton administration. In addition, key individuals were able to bridge the two networks, in particular, Nafis Sadiq, a Muslim woman who became Executive Director of UNFPA in 1987, and who was the organizer of the ICPD.

Thus, although conflict remained over how the new agenda was to be funded, there was some agreement within the donor community that it was time to reorient family-planning programmes away from population control and incorporate other areas of women's health. The United States Agency for International Development was already funding some HIV-related and maternal health programmes. Indeed, USAID funded maternal health activities through the MotherCare projects, despite lacking a congressional mandate, on the strength of advice by their technical staff, many of whom were women who identified with the aims of the women's movement. This shift also reflected evidence from elsewhere that health problems like HIV/STIs and maternal health (including abortion-related mortality) were of paramount importance, and that family-planning programmes could no longer ignore this public health context (Murphy and Merrick 1996). Along with evidence of the effectiveness of treating STIs at PHC levels for controlling HIV, this political consensus forged the new agenda for integrating HIV/STI services with family planning (Hardee and Yount 1995).

International co-operation at the conference itself

In sum, in the lead up to the ICPD, there were different issues driving family planning, maternal health, and HIV/STI policy. Yet many of the actors overlapped and used each other's arguments to bolster support for their specific positions. International family-planning policy had a much longer history of effort and a greater record of achievement than HIV or maternal health policy, although it was increasingly criticized. Maternal health programmes and policies had developed independently but with few resources and little success in reducing maternal death rates. International HIV policy also had very little success to boast of and, in the face of a devastating new pandemic, was searching for innovative approaches. This was reflected in international funding in 1990: of total external assistance to reproductive health services, 42 per cent went to population; 8 per cent to HIV/STIs, and a mere 0.2 per cent to safe motherhood (although a further 16 per cent went to MCH services which would mainly have targeted child health) (Zeitlin *et al.* 1994).

In this context, delegates from over 180 governments around the world met at the ICPD, accompanied by representatives of around 1200 international NGOs with interests from a wide range of contexts and ideologies (Sadasivam 1995; US Network for Cairo 1994). This was more than ten times the number of NGOs at the 1974 Bucharest Population Conference (Anonymous 1999) and the ICPD Programme of Action depicted an unprecedented consensus among women's groups, governments, and international agencies over the need to address reproductive ill health through re-orienting family planning away from meeting demographic targets and towards a primary level service designed to meet the needs of individual women (Lane 1994). This consensus was reaffirmed a year later at the Beijing Fourth World Conference on Women (UN 1995*a*; Cook and Fathalla 1996).

The package of reproductive health services for meeting these needs included: pre- and post-labour care plus obstetric management, contraception, prevention and management of reproductive tract infections (including HIV/STIs), abortion, reproductive cancer control, infertility treatment, and prevention of violence (McGinn *et al.* 1996). Service delivery strategies emphasized PHC approaches and an integrated (or supermarket approach to care). As a result, among international organizations, calls for integration became widespread (Pachauri 1994; Hardee and Yount 1995; USAID 1995; Mayhew 1996).

Almost immediately, however, the problems of moving from the rhetoric of a UN conference to the reality of service delivery in low-income country settings were acknowledged (Hardee and Yount 1995; International Council on Management of Population Programmes 1996). Lack of evidence for effectiveness or feasibility of many of the interventions advocated was seized on by a range of actors, including family planning providers, worried about loss of funds to broader reproductive health (Cleland 1996; Murphy and Merrick 1996; Potts and Walsh 1999); religious groups, opposed to contraceptive use or sexual rights (McIntosh and Finkle 1995); women's groups in low income countries, concerned about inappropriate application of health blueprints (Basu 1996; Basu 1997); and economists, with concerns about lack of adequate funds or analysis of financial implications (Finkle and McIntosh 1996; Conly and Epp 1997; Mitchell *et al.* 1999). Despite this substantial and varied dissent within large parts of the network which would be centrally involved in reproductive health, the concept was confirmed in the ICPD Programme of Action and commitments were made by international donors and national governments to fund relevant activities (Lane 1994).

However, while the international donor community claimed to support the approach and ideas of reproductive health strongly in the mid–1990s, its subsequent funding of relevant activities fell far short of commitments. For example, the total global annual cost of implementing the Programme of Action was estimated to be US$17 billion, of which two-thirds was to be met by national governments and one-third by donors. However, while governments came reasonably close to their commitments, donors met only small proportions of theirs: in 1996, the USA committed US$2.2 billion but gave US$640 million (29 per cent); the UK committed US$380 million but gave US$100 million (26 per cent); and Japan committed US$1.4 billion but gave a mere US$100 million (seven per cent) (Potts and Walsh 1999). Combined with their keen participation in the consensus at ICPD, these figures suggest that international donors were more committed to policy formulation than to its subsequent implementation.

Impact of ideology on reproductive health

The impacts of two ideologies, PHC and women's status, on development of policy in family planning, maternal health, HIV/STIs, and reproductive health can be seen at various points in time. In maternal health in the 1970s, it was thought that training TBAs could improve equity in access to health care; it is now recognized that it would be unlikely to reduce maternal mortality (Koblinsky *et al.* 1999). Moreover, in a constrained resource environment, the push by PHC to develop minimally trained multipurpose health workers led to a decrease in training of specialist cadres, those most necessary for preventing maternal deaths. For example, in the mid–1970s, the Bangladesh government discontinued training women who were in effect specialist community midwives and replaced them with family welfare visitors who were eventually to prioritize the delivery of contraceptives at the community level (Sherrat

1999). Similarly, in Egypt, midwifery schools were closed in the 1970s, and the current shortage of trained personnel with midwifery skills is a consequence that many other countries share today (Kwast 1992).

Equally, the women's movement advocated maternal health as part of women's health, yet showed a curious lack of interest in the details of obstetric care and the practicalities of achieving good services in this area. For example, a book on feminist perspectives on reproductive health makes only one mention of maternal mortality, and even that is about abortion, an area where the international women's movement has remained much more involved (Correa 1994). Women's groups were also fearful of focusing too much on women's traditional value as mothers, and this contributed to an uneasy relationship between women's health advocates and the SMI members. For their part, SMI advocates distanced themselves from the feminist agenda and attempted to focus on the technical aspects of safe motherhood, rather than diluting it by addressing women's status and living conditions more broadly: 'SMI is not the women's initiative. It is not intended to meet all of women's medical and social needs' (Law *et al.* 1991).

The ideology of the international women's movement was also a clear influence on the ICPD, as reflected in the Programme of Action. In Chapter II, principle four states (UN 1995*a*):

> advancing gender quality and equity and the empowerment of women, and the elimination of all kinds of violence against women, and ensuring women's ability to control their won fertility are cornerstones of population and development-related programmes. The human rights of women and the girl child are an inalienable, integral and indivisible part of human rights. . .

Chapter IV on 'Gender equality, equity and empowerment of women' recognizes the reduction of imbalances between women and men as an end in itself and as an essential element of sustainable development, for the first time in international population policy (Germain and Kyte 1995; Petchesky 1995). These aspects of the document reflected the efforts of the international women's movement to present a consensus on women's rights, despite major differences in their agenda. Differences were most marked between 'northern' and 'southern' feminists, who were concerned about sexual rights and sustainable development respectively, but who managed to hide their differences in order to maximize their influence on the outcome of the document (De Jong in press). As a result, even abortion is recognized as a service women have a right to (UN 1995*a*).

At the ICPD, however, the women's movement had to negotiate more directly with those promoting a PHC approach than they did over maternal health. This is seen clearly in the on-going debate over integration of HIV/STI services with family planning, where the ideological negotiations between these two groups led to a shift away from vertical family-planning programmes and towards a more comprehensive package of care. To justify the new approach, those drafting the ICPD Programme of Action absorbed many of the PHC concepts described above. Chapter VIII started with a discussion of PHC; In earlier chapters to improve reproductive health, governments committed to involve civil society (especially women's groups), to further programme design, to focus on prevention of reproductive ill health, and to promote a multi-sectoral approach (UN1995a). This apparently ignored 20 years of PHC experience, which suggested that a comprehensive approach was difficult to implement in practice, given low levels of funding (Walt and Vaughan 1982).

Furthermore, the publication of the Mwanza trial results in 1995 coincided neatly with the post-ICPD prioritization period and, in conjunction with the urgency of the HIV pandemic, led to a heavy emphasis on this area of reproductive health. During the confusion, the term 'integrated', usually referring to a limited combination of family planning with STI management, became synonymous with 'comprehensive' (Hardee and Yount 1995). This approach was convenient for family-planning policy makers, since it allowed them to claim progress on the ICPD agenda but involved minimal real change to existing policies and programmes (Mayhew *et al.* submitted for publication). Similarly, HIV/STI policy makers were satisfied since the approach gave them access to the superior international donor funds already allocated to family planning.

Policy development for integration was thus supported by an apparently highly effective new intervention against HIV (syndromic management of STIs) which fitted well with prevailing ideological paradigms (PHC emphasis and attention to women). However, in this case, as for maternal health, ideological imperatives masked practical reality: syndromic management of STIs *among women* is not very effective for controlling HIV. That this crucial piece of the jigsaw puzzle was missed in the post-ICPD and Mwanza trial euphoria suggests that something more than scientific imperatives drove policy makers.

Lessons for the future

During 30 years of reproductive health policy development there have been significant disjunctures between the networks and ideologies of actors involved in international policy decisions, which have negatively affected policy impact. Analysing the processes of international negotiation and co-operation is therefore important for furthering our understanding of how ideology can be better used to support rather than hinder policy developments. There are two principal lessons for future international co-operative efforts.

(1) International actors bring specific interests to the table, often related to macro-level political or economic ideology, and their negotiations can drive shifts in global policy agendas very rapidly.

(2) Despite good intentions, technical public-health detail often gets lost in the translation from international ideologically driven rhetoric to practical application in programme design, funding, and service algorithms.

Global networks of policy makers that form around particular issues are often transient and founded on convenient allegiances between actors with radically different ideologies and priorities. In establishing consensus and co-operation, rapid progress can be achieved in determining new policy approaches, which can have a positive effect. However, in understanding these networks, few studies have addressed in detail the roles of different types of actors, including communities of technical experts or media/public relations groups. Our findings suggest that the absence of a complementary coalition of such actors around a specific health issue leaves that issue vulnerable to the whims of less well-informed and more ideological groups.

Secondly, while these groups may be aware of the unrealistic nature of their agreements, the process of negotiation and achieving consensus can lead them to lose sight of feasibility. Again, this might be avoided by greater representation of the views of national representatives or technical experts at international events. Bringing such a 'reality check' back into international fora should not obliterate the potential for radical policy change, which can be a good thing in itself, but should perhaps aim to temper optimism and deliver more helpful programmes for action.

Acknowledgements

The research on which this chapter is based was supported by UK DFID under their 'Improving People's Benefit from Reproductive Health Services' and 'Effective Services, Effective Policies: New Knowledge for Safer Motherhood in Poor Countries' research programmes. We would also like to thank Jelka Zupan for her helpful comments on an earlier draft.

References

AbouZahr, C. (1998) Maternal mortality overview. In *Health dimensions of sex and reproduction*, ed. C. J. L. Murray and A. D. Lopez. Harvard University Press, Boston.

Adler, M., Foster, S., Grosskurth *et al.* (1998) Sexual health and health care: sexually transmitted infections. Guidelines for prevention and treatment. Health and population Occasional Paper. Department for International Development: London.

Agarwal, B. (1994) The gender and environment debate: lessons from India In *Population and environment: rethinking the debate*, ed. L. Arizpe, M. P. Stone, and D. C. Major. Westview Press, Boulder.

Ainsworth, M. and Over, A. M. (1994) The economic impact of AIDS in Africa In *AIDS in Africa*, ed. M. Essex, S. Mboup, P. J. Kanki *et al.* Raven Press, New York.

Anonymous (1999) UN assesses the success of ICPD. *Population Today,* **27**(1), 4–5.

Ashford, L. (1995) Implementing reproductive health programmes. Report of a donor workshop co-sponsored by the UK Overseas Development Administration and the US Agency for International Development, 12–14 June, New York. London School of Hygiene and Tropical Medicine, London.

Backett, E. M., Davies, A. M., and Petros-Barvazian (1984) The risk approach in health care, with special reference to maternal and child health including family planning. *Public Health Papers,* **76**, 1–113.

Basu, A. M. (1996) ICPD: What about men's rights and women's responsibilities. *Health Transition Review*, **6**(2), 225–7.

Basu, A. M. (1997) The new international population movement: a framework for a constructive critique. *Health Transition Review,* **7**(Suppl. 4), 7–32.

Behets, F. M., Williams, Y., Braithwaite, A. *et al* (1995) Management of vaginal discharge in women treated at a Jamaican sexually transmitted disease clinic: use of diagnostic algorithms versus laboratory testing. *Clinical Infectious Disease,* **21**(6), 1450–5.

Belsey, M. A. (1985) Traditional birth attendants: a resource for the health of women. *International Journal of Gynecology and Obstetrics*, **23**(4), 247–8.

Bergstrom, S., Molin, A., and Povey, G. W. (1992) International maternal health care 1992, the challenge beyond the year 2000. Department of Obstetrics and Gynecology, Uppsala University.

Berman, P. (1995) *Health sector reform in developing countries*. Harvard University Press, Boston.

Bloom, D. E. and Godwin, P. The economics of HIV and AIDS: the case of south and south east Asia. Oxford University Press, Delhi.

Bose, A. (1989) India's quest for population stabilisation: progress, pitfalls and policy options. *Demography India*, **18**(1–2), 261–73.

Boserup, E. (1989) Population, the status of women and rural development. In *Rural development population (supplement to Population and Development Review)*, ed. G. McNicoll and M. Cain. Population Council, New York.

Caldwell, J. C., Orubuloye, I. O., and Caldwell, P. (1992) Underreaction to AIDS in Sub-Saharan Africa. *Social Science and Medicine*, **34**, 1169–82.

Chen, L. C. (1986) Primary health care in developing countries: overcoming operation, technical, and social barriers. *Lancet*, **2**(8518), 1260–5.

Cleland, J. (1996) ICPD and the feminization of population and development issues. *Health Transition Review*, **6**(1), 107–10.

Cohen, M. S. (1998) Sexually transmitted diseases enhance HIV transmission: no longer a hypothesis. *Lancet* **351** (Suppl. III), S1115–S1117.

Collins, C. and Green, A. (1994) Decentralization and primary health care: some negative implications in developing countries. *International Journal of Health Services*, **24**(3), 459–75.

Conly, S. R. and Epp, J. E. (1997) *Falling short: the World Bank's role in population and reproductive health*. Population Action International, Washington DC.

Cook, R. J. and Fathalla, M. F. (1996) Advancing reproductive rights beyond Cairo and Beijing. *International Family Planning Perspectives*, **22**(3), 115–21.

Correa, S. S. (1994) *Population and reproductive rights feminist perspectives from the south*. Zed Books, New Delhi.

De Cock, K. M., Ekpini, E., Gnaore, E. *et al.* (1994) The public health implications of AIDS research in Africa. *Journal of the American Medical Association*, **272**, 481–6.

Dejong, J. (in press) The role and limitations of the Cairo International Conference on Population and Development. *Social Science and Medicine.*

Delay, P. (1998) Presentation on USAID and AIDS. Setting the African Agenda II Conference. Nairobi.

Finkle, J. L. and McIntosh, A. (1994) *The new politics of population: conflict and concensus in family planning. population and development review*. The Population Council, New York.

Finkle, J. L. and McIntosh, A. (1996) Cairo revisited: some thoughts on the implications of the ICPD. *Health Transition Review*, **6**(1), 111–3.

Folbre, N. (1983) Of patriarchy born: the political economy of fertility decisions. *Feminist Studies*, **9**, 84.

Folbre, N. (1992) "The improper arts": sex in classical political economy. *Population and Development Review*, **18**(1), 105–21, 205–8.

Garcia-Moreno, C. and Claro, A. (1994) Challenges from the women's health movement: women's rights versus population control. In *Population policies reconsidered: health empowerment and rights*, ed. G. Sen, A. Germain and L. C. Chen. Harvard Center for Population and Development, Boston.

Gerbase, A. C., Rowley, J. T., and Mertens, T. E. (1998) Global epidemiology of sexually transmitted disease. *Lancet*, 351 (Suppl. III), SIII2–SIII4.

Germain, A. (1987) Reproductive health and dignity: choices by third world women. *International Conference on Better Health for Women and Children through Family Planning*. International Women's Health Coalition, Nairobi/New York.

Germain, A. and Kyte, R. (1995) *The Cairo consensus: the right agenda for the right time*. International Women's Health Coalition, New York.

Gilson, L., Mkanje, R., Frosskurth, H. *et al.* (1997) Cost-effectiveness of improved treatment services for sexually transmitted diseases in preventing HIV–1 infection in Mwanza Region, Tanzania. *Lancet*, 350, 1805–9.

Graham, W. J. and Campbell, O. M. R. (1990) Measuring maternal health: defining the issues. Maternal and child epidemiology unit report. London School of Hygiene and Tropical Medicine, London.

Grosskurth, H. (1999) From Mwanza and Rakai to Beijing and Moscow? STD Control and HIV prevention. *Sexually Transmitted Infections*, 75, 83–9.

Grosskurth, H. F., Mosha, F., Todd, J. *et al.* (1995) Impact of improved treatment of sexually transmitted diseases on HIV infection in rural Tanzania:randomised control trial. *Lancet*, 346, 530–6.

Hardee, K. and Yount, K. M. (1995) *From rhetoric to reality: delivering reproductive health promises through integrated services*. Family Health International, Research Triangle Park, North Carolina.

Hartmann, B. (1987) *Reproductive rights and wrongs: the global politics of population control*. Harper and Row, New York.

Hawkes, S., Morison, L., Foster, S. *et al* (1999) Reproductive-tract infections in women in low-income, low prevalence situations: assessment of syndromic management in Matlab, Bangladesh. *Lancet*, 354(9192), 1776–81.

Hayes, R., Grosskurth, H., and Ka-Gina, G. (1995) Impact of improved treatment of sexually transmitted disease on HIV infection. *Lancet*, 346, 1159–60.

Hesketh, T. and Zhu, W. X. (1997) Health in China. The one child family policy: the good, the bad, and the ugly. *British Medical Journal*, 314(7095), 1685–7.

Holmes, K. K. and Ryan, C. A. (1999) STD care management. In *Sexually Transmitted Diseases*, ed. S. K. K. Holme, P. F. Sparling, P. A. Mardh *et al*. McGraw-Hill, London.

International Council on Management of Population Programmes (1996) Managing quality reproductive health programmes: after Cairo and beyond. Report of an international seminar. International Council on Management of Population Programmes, Addis Ababa.

International Labour Organisation (1995) The impact of HIV/AIDS on the productive labour force in Africa. EAMAT Working Paper Number 1. International Labour Organisation, Addis Ababa.

Jain, A., Bruce, J., and Mensch, B. (1992) Setting standards of quality in family planning programs. *Studies in Family Planning*, 23(6 Part 1), 392–5.

Janovsky, K. (1996) *Health policy and systems development: an agenda for research*. WHO, Geneva.

Kabeer, N. (1994) *Reversed realities: gender hierarchies in development thought.* Verso Books, London.

Kalumba, K. (1997) Towards an equity-oriented policy of decentralization in health systems under conditions of turbulence: the case of Zambia. Forum on Health Sector Reform, WHO, Geneva.

Koblinsky, M. A., Campbell, O. M. R., and Heichelheim, J. (1999) Organizing delivery care: what works for safe motherhood? *Bulletin of the World Health Organisation,* **77**(5), 399–406.

Kwast, B. E. (1992) Midwives: key rural health workers in maternity care. *International Journal of Gynecology and Obstetrics,* **38** (June Suppl.), S9–S15.

Lane, S. D. (1994) From population control to reproductive health: an emerging policy agenda. *Social Science and Medicine,* **39**(9), 1303–14.

Law, M., Maine, D., and Feuerstein, M. T. (1991) Safe motherhood, priorities and next steps forward looking assessment on the reduction of maternal motality and morbidity within the framework of the SMI. UNDP.

Lee, K. and Walt, G. (1995) Linking national and global population agendas: case studies from eight developing countries. *Third World Quarterly,* **16**(2), 257–72.

Lee, K. and Zwi, A. (1996) A global political economy approach to AIDS; ideology, interests and implications. *New Political Economy,* **1**(3), 355–73.

Loudon, I. (1992) *Death in childbirth: an international study of maternal care and maternal mortality, 1800–1960.* Clarendon Press, Oxford.

Lucas, A. (1997) History of the prevention of maternal mortality network. *International Journal of Gynecology and Obstetrics,* **59**(November Suppl. 2), S11–S14.

Mahler, H. (1987) The safe motherhood initiative; a call to action. *The Lancet,* **1**(8534) 668–70.

Maine, D. (1991) Safe motherhood programs: options and issues. Center for Population and Family Health, School of Public Health, Faculty of Medicine, Columbia University, New York.

Mayaud, P. (2000) Personal communication. London School of Hygiene and Tropical Medicine.

Mayhew, S. (1996) Integrating MCH/FP and STD/HIV services: current debates and future directions. *Health Policy and Planning,* **11**(4), 339–53.

Mayhew, S., Walt, G., Lush, L. *et al.* (submitted for publication) Donor involvement in reproductive health: saying one thing and doing another? *Health Policy and Planning.*

McGinn, T., Maine, D., McCarthy, K. *et al.* (1996) Setting priorities in international reproductive health programs: a practical framework. Centre for Population and Family Health, Columbia School of Public Health, New York.

McIntosh, C. A. and Finkle, J. L. (1995) The Cairo conference on population and development: a new paradigm? *Population and Development Review,* **21**(2), 223–60.

McPake, B., Hanson, K., and Mills, A. (1993) Community financing of health care in Africa: an evaluation of the Mamako initiative. *Social Science and Medicine,* **36**(11), 1383–95.

Mitchell, M. D., Littlefield, J., and Gutter, S. (1999) Costing of reproductive health services. *International Family Planning Perspectives,* **25** (Suppl.), S17–S21.

Murphy, E. and Merrick, T. (1996) Did "Cairo" delete "population" from population policy? Washington DC, PATH and the World Bank.

Oppenheim Mason, K. (1993) The impact of women's social position on fertility in developing countries. In *Demography as an interdiscipline,* ed. J. Sytycos. Transaction, Oxford.

Over, M. (1998) Coping with the impact of AIDS. *Finance and Development,* 1998(March), 22–4.

Pachauri, S. (1994) Relationship between AIDS and FP programmes: a rationale for developing integrated reproductive health services. *Health Transition Review,* 4(Suppl.: AIDS impact and prevention in the developing world: demographic and social science perspectives).

Petchesky, R. P. (1995) From population control to reproductive rights: feminist fault lines. *Reproductive Health Matters,* 6, 152–61.

Potts, M. and Walsh, J. (1999) Making Cairo work. *Lancet,* 353, 315–18.

Reich, M. R. (1995) The politics of agenda setting in international health: child health versus adult health in developing countries. *Journal of International Development,* 7(3), 489–502.

Rifkin, S. B. and Walt, G. (1986) Why health improves: defining the issues concerning 'comprehensive primary health care' and 'selective primary health care'. *Social Science and Medicine,* 23(6), 559–66.

Rooney, C. I. F. (1992) Antenatal care and maternal health: how effective is it? WHO/MSM/92.4. WHO, Geneva.

Rosenfield, A. and Maine, D. (1985) Maternal mortality – a neglected tragedy. Where is the M in MCH? *The Lancet,* 2, 83–5.

Ross, J. A., Maudlin, S. W., Green, S. R. *et al.* (1992) *Family planning and child survival programs (as assessed in 1991).* The Population Council, New York.

Ryan, C. A., Zidhough, A., Manhart, L. E. *et al.* (1998) Reproductive tract infections in primary healthcare, family planning and dermatovenereology clinics: evaluation of syndromic management in Morocco. *Sexually Transmitted Infections,* 74 (Suppl. 1), S95–S105.

Sadasivam, B. (1995) NGOs on ICPD: "Keep your promises". *Populi,* 22(4), 6–7.

Sen, G., Germain, A. and Chen, L. C. (1994) *Population policies reconsidered: health empowerment rights.* Harvard School of Public Health, Boston.

Sherrat, D. R. (1999) Why women need midwives for safe motherhood. In *Reproductive health matters. Safe motherhood initiatives: critical issues,* ed. M. Berer and T. K. S. Ravindran. Blackwell Science, Oxford.

Shulman, C., Dorman E. K., Cutts, F., Kawuondo, K., Bulmer, J., Peshu, N. & Marsh, K. (1999). Preventing severe anaemia secondary to malaria in pregnancy: a double blind randomized placebo control trial of sulphadoxine-pyrimethamine. *Lancet* 353(9153): 632–636.

Taylor, C. E., Newman, J. S., and Kelly, N. U. (1976) The child survival hypothesis. *Population Studies,* 30(2), 263–78.

UNAIDS (1998a) *AIDS Epidemic Update: December 1998.* UNAIDS and WHO, Geneva.

UNAIDS (1998b) Report on the global HIV/AIDS epidemic: June 1998. UNAIDS and WHO, Geneva.

UNAIDS (1999) *AIDS Epidemic Update: December 1999.* UNAIDS and WHO, Geneva.

UN (1995a) Population and development. Vol. 1, Programme of action adopted at the International Conference on Population and Development, Cairo, 5–13 September 1994. Department for Economic and Social Information and Policy Analysis, UN, New York.

UN (1995b) Report of the Fourth World Conference on Women, Beijing, 4–15 September 1995. FWCW Secretariat/Division of the Advancement of Women, UN, New York.

US Network for Cairo (1994) Consensus reached on watershed document at ICPD. *Cairo '94,* **1**(7), 1–2.

USAID (1995) Setting the African agenda: final report on a workshop on integration of HIV/AIDS with MCH/FP in Nairobi. USAID Regional Office for Eastern and Southern Africa, Nairobi.

van Stavaren, I. (1994) A political economy of reproduction. *Development* , **3**, 20–3.

Vaughan, J. P. (1987) Background discussion paper for the Steering Committee meeting of the safe motherhood operational research (SMOR) programme. 13–14 July 1987. WHO, Geneva.

Walt, G. (1998) Globalisation of international health. *Lancet,* **351**(9100), 434–37.

Walt, G. and Vaughan, P. (1982) Primary health care: what does it mean? *Tropical Doctor,* **12**(3), 99–100.

Wasserheit, J. N. (1992) Epidemiological synergy: interrelationships between human immunodeficiency virus infection and other sexually transmitted diseases. *Sexually Transmitted Diseases,* **19**(2), 61–77.

Westoff, C. F. and Ochoa, L. H. (1991) *Unmet need and the demand for family planning.* Macro International, Maryland.

WHO (1974) Health and family planning. Working Paper No. 136, World Population Conference. WHO, Geneva.

WHO (1978). *International Conference on Primary Health Care: Alma Ata.* WHO/UNICEF, Geneva.

WHO (1991) Essential elements of obstetric care at the first referral leval. WHO, Geneva.

WHO (1996) Revised 1990 estimates of maternal mortality. A new approach by WHO and UNICEF. WHO/FRH/MSM/96.11.

WHO (1999) World health report 1999: making a difference. WHO, Geneva.

WHO/GPA (1995) Global prevalence and incidences of selected curable sexually transmitted diseases: overview and estimates. *WHO/GPA/STD,* **1**, 1–26.

World Bank (1993) *World development report: investing in health.* Oxford University Press, Oxford.

World Federation of Public Health Associations (1986) Women and health. Information for action issue paper. World Federation of Public Health Associations, Geneva.

Zapata, B. C. and Godue, C. J. M. (1997) International maternal and child health. In *Maternal and child health: programs, problems and policy in public health,* ed. J. B. Kotch. Aspen, Gaithersburg, Maryland.

Zeitlin, J., Govindaraj, R., and Chen, L. (1994) Financing reproductive and sexual health services. In *Population policies reconsidered: health, empowerment and rights,* ed. G. Sen, A. Germain, and L. C. Chen. Harvard Center for Population and Development Studies, Harvard University, Boston, Massachusetts.

Chapter 11

The way forward

Paul Garner and Martin McKee

The challenges

Even if the word is not explicitly used, the effects of globalization appear every day in our newspapers and on our television screens as we are constantly reminded of how the world is shrinking. But as the preceding 10 chapters make clear, globalization is an extremely complex phenomenon. On the one hand, the images of its effects on the lives of ordinary people, whether they are car workers in the UK, caribou herders in Alaska, or farmers in Burundi are clear. But we face many challenges when we try to quantify these consequences. How many lives are ended prematurely? How much additional disability is created? Does the imagery of crisis obscure the less news-worthy benefits that globalization brings? And how can we be sure that what we are seeing is really the consequence of global phenomena?

We have sought in this book to highlight a few aspects of globalization, looking at their impact on health. But where does this analysis take us, as informed professionals concerned about the world around us?

What emerges over and over again is that the health-related consequences of glob-alization most often appear in terms of threats. We see these clearly in the chapters on global trade, military spending, and the damage to the ecosystem. The opportunities may be there but they are currently less easy to find.

This negative imagery could be dismissed simply as a consequence of the changing nature of news presentation. The benefits of technological progress are more difficult to capture on video in a way that can compete with the graphic images of wars and other disasters that are now beamed into our homes in real time. The demands on politicians and others for instant responses gives little time for reflection on how threats could be turned into opportunities. But there is also a more fundamental problem, which lies at the heart of the process of globalization. Although superficially it is about a world of advancing technology and increasing wealth, fundamentally, as we have seen in Chapters 1 and 2, it is characterized by shifts in power, away from individuals and from the governments that represent them. A major achievement of the twentieth century was the global spread of democracy. This was hailed as a means of giving power to the people, exercised through their elected representatives. But by the 1990s, when democracy was spreading across the Soviet bloc and Africa, politi-cians were increasingly constrained in their ability to influence events around them. The challenges they faced were trans-national but the tools available to them were increasingly constrained by their national boundaries.

A new global environment has now arrived that is much more complex than the one it has replaced. What is more, it is here to stay and there is no going back. Governments have long recognized the need for international co-operation, in all sorts of areas. In Chapter 1 we traced the developments that led to the creation of the World Health Organization (WHO). As one of the United Nations (UN) specialized agencies it was based on a particular model of international co-operation, in which states interacted vertically with international agencies (Walt 2001). The new global environment encompasses many more types of actors: sub-national governments, supra-national regional bodies (such as the European Union), private industry, non-governmental organizations (NGOs), universities, and even some individuals, such as the major philanthropists. This environment is, however, somewhat chaotic. There is no overarching global integration, no new world order, no unifying global structure, and little democratic accountability.

This process is generating some new trans-national structures but these have proved highly controversial. The World Trade Organization (WTO) offers a means for governments to create a set of rules for global commerce. On the one hand, some see the process of globalization, guided by the appropriate rules, as offering the potential to reduce world poverty. They argue that structures may be imperfect but it is important to be at the coal face, contributing to the agenda and making things work for the public good (Secretary for State for International Development 1999).

Others argue that the process of globalization and the structures associated with it, and in particular the WTO, are flawed and will simply entrench existing divisions of power to make the richer nations more powerful, at the expense of the poor and less well developed (Pollock and Price 2000). When a country does not even have the resources to maintain a permanent representation in Geneva it is difficult for it to make its voice heard; and as Lang notes, in Chapter 6, especially at technical discussions, the national delegations from some industrialized countries have essentially been hijacked by trans-national corporate interests.

The complex arguments about the 'good' and 'bad' sides of globalization will continue, but what is clear is that these power shifts will result in winners and losers (Walt 1998). As globalization gives national governments less control of what happens within their borders, so they must engage in new structures and networks that will allow them to act collectively to minimize the threats to health that globalization brings, at the same time as maximizing the opportunities that it offers. Governments have a responsibility to listen to a wider range of interests and to involve new actors, in particular from civil society. As health professionals, we have a responsibility to help this process.

In this concluding chapter we revisit some of the threats that are posed to the public health by globalization and we explore some of the opportunities it offers, in particular, how health professionals can come together to promote global public health.

The threats to health

The growth in global trade has undoubtedly brought many benefits to many people. This has generated an enthusiasm among many politicians, especially in the leading industrialized nations, to accelerate the process by removing remaining barriers to trade. By doing so, they believe, wealth will increase and, even if it does not immediately flow to the poor, it will ultimately trickle down to them, eventually enhancing their health and well-being.

Unfortunately past examples give little cause for such optimism. Free trade is unlikely to improve health if what is being traded is harmful. Many governments accept this argument, spending vast amounts to restrict trade in narcotics. It was not always so, of course, and the UK grew rich from cultivation of opium in India in the nineteenth century, which they then sold to the Chinese (Wong 1998). Any threat to this 'free trade' was met by military intervention. While western governments no longer promote free trade in narcotics, they have less compunction about other goods that are equally lethal. In Chapter 7, Holdstock points out that global investment in arms is around US$700 billion per annum. There are thus powerful vested interests in maintaining global production and trade in goods designed to kill whole populations.

Conversion to investment in public goods that actually benefit the public makes sense, but how will more liberal trading arrangements between nations contribute to this? Since 1945 most deaths from armed conflict have been amongst the world's poor, and these countries are key markets for western arms companies (Sidel 1995). Here, it appears, control needs to be tightened, not loosened. Wipfli and colleagues demonstrate the damage done by global trade in tobacco and, with an enviable sense of optimism, propose that the new framework convention on tobacco control will address the rise and spread of tobacco consumption. Kickbusch and Buse have noted the similarity in the campaigns waged by the arms and tobacco industries against regulation that might restrict their markets, in both cases with major implications for the harm that is done to children (Kickbusch and Buse 2001).

It is not only trade in goods that are actually harmful. In any transaction, the strong will more often triumph over the weak. Global trade is often a very unequal struggle, between trans-national corporations on the one hand and small local producers on the other. Some countries are in a much better position than others to benefit from global opening of markets, for many different reasons, some of which have their origins far in the past (Landes 1998). Attempts to redress the balance, by forming co-operatives or establishing fair trade arrangements, are often met by tactics ranging from predatory pricing to physical violence. The established hierarchies are reinforced by the partial nature of freedom of movement on offer in the world economic order. Free movement of goods and capital are not accompanied by free movement of labour, except for a small global elite. Executives decide where they will invest, produce goods (and increasingly services, via the internet and telephone call centres), where they live, and where they pay taxes but their workers do not have the same choices. Any attempt to exercise such a choice will label them as 'economic migrants' thus ranking them below political refugees on the list of unwanted visitors.

Finally, the transactions involved in global trade frequently fail to take account of all of the costs, which may be borne by future generations. Trans-national trade in food can damage fragile local economies in deprived areas of the world, and, as Lang points out, is unlikely to have any impact on reducing hunger among the poor. Furthermore, the ecological damage created by unregulated development, such as deforestation, makes communities much more vulnerable to the effects of an increasingly unstable climate.

Of course the outlook for poor countries is not entirely pessimistic. Recently an Indian company, Tata tea bought out Tetley for US$370 million, and Indian entrepreneurs are emerging as global players. In this case, globalization seems to be turning imperialism on its head (Kutumbakam 2000). Such examples are, however, rare.

The needs

Ecological problems need global responses

We live in a world where an increasing population continually strives for higher standards of living. This has two different but related elements. One is the damage done by the massive ecological footprints left by the rich as they seek an even higher standard of living. At least as important are the consequences arising from the struggle by the poor to achieve living standards that the rest of us already have. The environment suffers not only from the excessive demands placed on it by affluence, but also the destruction caused by poverty. People in poorer regions are forced to accept destruction of their own lands simply because they are disempowered. This lack of power also prevents them from challenging poorly controlled industrial development, exemplified by the circumstances surrounding the toxic chemical disaster at Bhopal. McMichael and Woodward, in Chapter 5, highlight the irony that the most vulnerable to environmental change are the impoverished as they have fewer choices at their disposal.

The scale of global inequity makes it difficult for those in the west to demand that the developing world constrain its development to preserve the global environment. It is clear that ecological problems will require global responses, but they will need extraordinary levels of collective action. The 'cosmopolitan consciousness' needed to take this forward is problematic as this is a threat with no frontiers, and as communities and nations we are used to the dialectic of enemy images (Beck 2000). In fact, the enemy is within ourselves, whether we are the rich wanting more, or the poor trying to move out of their position of disadvantage.

Disease control needs global mechanisms

Globalization brings threats to public health from infectious diseases. As we noted in Chapter 1, trade historically has helped to spread syphilis, plague, and smallpox, among others. Chirimuuta has argued persuasively that trade has spread human immunodeficiency virus (HIV) throughout Africa, demonstrated by its spread from ports, urban centres, and truck routes into the body of the continent (Chirimuuta 1989). Today, travel helps the spread of pandemics of influenza, and continues to exacerbate the problems of the spread of tuberculosis (TB) and sexually transmitted diseases. Increased spread of microbial resistant organisms, such as malaria, tuberculosis, and gonorrhoea increase suffering and make treatment more complicated and expensive.

The sheer volume of regional and global responses outlined by Weinberg in Chapter 4 suggest that we do not yet have effective mechanisms for monitoring or control of the spread of disease globally. Options open to national governments acting alone, such as compulsory health checks for migrants, will have little impact on the spread of disease. These threats need global responses, and, at a very minimum, global mechanisms for surveillance and investigation of outbreaks. Yet systems remain fragmentary. In particular, the ability to identify patterns of microbial drug resistance is poorly developed. Many of the threats posed by infectious diseases in the fourteenth century remain: some of the diseases are different but the challenges have grown as mobility has increased.

The opportunities

The preceding section, with its litany of global threats and little evidence of effective action makes depressing reading. As Beck points out, the dangers of globalization are like negative currency. We know they are there but no-one wants to accept responsibility for them. But we should not lose sight of the opportunities associated with globalization, and it is these opportunities that provide potential mechanisms to help collectively tackle these problems. This book is about what health professionals can do to tackle these threats. Box 11.1 highlights four principles for action.

Box 11.1: Principles for health professionals in tackling threats to health arising from globalization

♦ aim to maximize the opportunities that globalization brings, for everyone

♦ strive to detect and quantify the health problems arising from globalization and to identify possible remedies

♦ assume that globalization is too important an issue to be left to the global capital markets – we all have a part to play

♦ believe that we can make a difference

A global approach to need and development

One positive aspect of a global view of the world is that it encourages collective thinking, mitigating against isolationism and nationalism in confronting problems of society and the environment. Most governments have seen health from a national or regional perspective. Globalization forces us to think of health need in a global sense, often graphically in television images of famines and environmental disasters. In doing so it compels us to seek ways to address inequities in health between nations. This has profound consequences for policies to tackle global inequity. Suddenly, the health of people in other countries is a legitimate concern. Simply voicing the concept of responsibility for health of people in other nations can have a profound effect on the way we see ourselves. It becomes easier to justify collaborative efforts to do something to redress global inequities.

A global view of need thus implies a global approach to find common solutions, with global networks that aim for globalization to benefit all and not just the already wealthy. One example is the way that the UK government has embraced this concept, creating a strategy for global development in the fight against poverty.

Communication and information

Advances in communications technology, in particular via the Internet, offer massive opportunities for improving information flow and generating global knowledge.

Wider access to information and knowledge can contribute to reductions in inequalities between individuals, groups, and countries. Knowledge is increasingly recognized as the third input into economic growth, alongside labour and capital (Braverman 1974). The technology that can enhance the spread of information globally already exists. Some governments and NGOs have already done much to put in place the infrastructure, such as the major investment by the Open Society Institute in a fibre-optic and satellite network linking Russian universities.

There are important new developments in the assimilation of research evidence about the benefits and harms of health care interventions, viewing research as a global resource in need of synthesis using good science (Cochrane Handbook 2001). New publishing ventures seek free access to medical literature, and Biomed Central is a welcome new initiative promoting free web access to medical research (Delamothe and Smith 2001).

Access to information can be incredibly empowering, which is why a few countries continue to try to restrict it. But political censorship is not the only threat. Another is the increasing privatization of knowledge under laws governing intellectual property rights. Stiglitz has argued persuasively for a regime that balances incentives for private generation of knowledge with the needs of society, and for the removal of existing barriers to the dissemination of publicly funded knowledge generation (Stiglitz 1999). But perhaps the main threat is the uneven access to the global information system. Africa, with 20 per cent of the world's population, has 2 per cent of the world's telephone lines and, while Internet access is expanding rapidly, it is still much more expensive than in industrialized countries (Sy 1999).

In the field of health, information technology is helping global compilations of sources of information, whether they are global statistics about health status, or summaries of benefits and harms of health care interventions that draw on the global literature. This is helping to democratize health knowledge, reducing the asymmetry of information between health professionals and the public. Knowledge becomes a cosmopolitan resource, drawn together irrespective of the country and setting, to highlight what does and does not work. This does, however, have a flip side: knowledge about health, disease, and what to do about it must be adapted to local circumstances. Thus, the determinants of certain diseases in one population may be less important in another (McKee *et al.* 2001) and a treatment that will be appropriate in one setting may not be in another. Practitioners and consumers need skills in interpreting global information in their own context.

Global influence

Lee has described the jurisdictional gap between the globalized world and national governments. Authors of several chapters describe the formal organizations and alliances that are developing to fill this gap. In Chapter 8, Wipfli and colleagues describe the WHO's efforts in tobacco control; in Chapter 5 McMichael and Woodward describe multi-disciplinary groups working on global changes co-ordinated through the UN Environmental Programme; Lush and Campbell, in Chapter 10, describe co-operation between the WHO, the World Bank, the UN Population Fund, and others in promoting basic rights in reproductive health; and Lang, in Chapter 6, explores the work of the WTO. Elsewhere, Lee has considered carefully the options for global health co-operation through global – predominantly UN-structures – with proposals for reform of the UN with wider participation to avoid the 'same old faces' and with a clear purpose and direction (Lee 1998).

All of these bodies are having to confront the issue of global governance raised in Chapter 1. While this is key to developing the structures required, it does not, however, help the concerned health professional identify whether they have a role to play. But they do, and they can, partly as a result of the nature of globalization itself. The process of globalization is creating global lobbies: social groups with common interests across nations, with common goals in advocating change. These groups are powerful forces with long tentacles and links into many systems and regions. Their power lies in the very roots of globalization.

If we accept there is no single global logic driving change, then globalization becomes a series of related phenomena with different drivers and influences. Put simplistically, economic globalization is about capitalists maximizing profit; technological globalization is about convergence of systems; and political globalization is about nations forming common agendas and military alliances. This then gives rise to transnational organizations working across communities of states, each with competing aims. These can be commercial organizations, political structures, professional groups, or informal networks.

In the absence of an overarching global political process, networks of individuals established through horizontal affiliation of people with common interests can influence the international political milieu around global concerns. International non-government campaigning agencies, such as Amnesty International, Greenpeace, and Oxfam have had considerable successes, working across national boundaries; and in Chapter 7, Holdstock notes how the International Physicians for Prevention of Nuclear War exerted a major influence on the progress of the nuclear arms race in the 1980s. Similar organizations (sometimes called 'civil societies') have had some spectacular successes in developing countries, including action on marketing of baby milk and on female genital mutilation. Debt relief, although already on several countries' agendas, was helped by Jubilee 2000, a coalition of over 90 organizations demanding for the world's poorest nations debt to be cancelled (Abbasi 1999). Drawing on the successes to date, protagonists are advocating a wider agenda for such groups, to tackle corruption, pollution, and imposed macro-economic policies that worsen poverty (Jareg and Kaseje 1998).

The contribution of health professionals

The purpose of this book was to advocate to health professionals that they need to be interested in the changes happening around them; that we need to look beyond our own parochial national interest as, increasingly, public health problems and solutions have to be considered in a global context.

How individuals do this will vary. As McMichael and Woodward argue persuasively in Chapter 5, one way is to promote and undertake a programme of research that will quantify the scale and scope of global influences on health. This will not be easy. So far, epidemiologists have tended to study exposures that are relatively easy to measure, such as cholesterol levels or smoking. Other exposures that are more difficult to measure, such as changes in weather, diet, or frequency (rather than average amount) of alcohol consumption, have received much less attention. In the area of globalization, where the exposures of interest are the effects of international trade, climate change, war, and civil disorder, or even genetically modified food, the challenges are enormous. In these cases, the chains of causation are often complex and obscure, demanding new epidemiological methods. Furthermore, those that may be most affected by globalization may not 'officially' exist in that only about 20 per cent of the world's population 'officially' exist, that is, their birth or death will be recorded by someone. Thus those most vulnerable to the effects of globalization are those of whom we know least. The challenges are magnified by the efforts of vested interests, of which the tobacco (Glantz *et al.* 1996) and asbestos (Tweedale 2000) industries are the best documented, to undermine the efforts of those promoting health and to spread disinformation (Box 11.2) (Ong and Glantz 2000). There is, however, a danger of the perfect becoming the enemy of the good and it will be essential for researchers to address these issues if they are to relevant in the twenty-first century. Quite simply, they must make the invisible visible.

Undertaking the research is only one challenge. The information must then be communicated to the public in a clear and comprehensible way. To do so effectively, however, researchers must also work to regain the trust that, in many countries, they have lost in recent years (McKee 1999). To do so they must ensure absolute transparency about potential conflict of interest; they must understand the complex nature of the concept of risk (Bernstein 1996; McKee 1999); and they must adopt a holistic perspective that takes account of the wider implications of particular issues. Thus, a debate on the effects of genetically modified foods is incomplete if it only examines their safety when fed to laboratory animals. It must also reflect the economic implications for those who produce the relevant foodstuff and for biodiversity.

Health professionals thus need to seize the opportunities for better health through research and development. The tools are available to monitor disease globally: why are we not seeking ways to predict outbreaks, and take pre-emptive action? We know drug resistance is a rapidly emerging problem: why are we not working globally to tackle this problem? The WHO shows some technical leadership in these areas, but

Box 11.2: **The tobacco industry and passive smoking: the International Agency for Research on Cancer (IARC) study**

Industry adopted a three-point strategy

Scientific

◆ industry lawyers identifying direction of research and commissioning research to 'confound' it

Communication

◆ promotion of 'good epidemiology practice', which would make epidemiological research prohibitively difficult and which would, specifically, discount relative risks less than two, which would thus exclude the typical values found for the health effects of environmental tobacco exposure

◆ selective leaking of initial results pre-publication to ensure the actual paper was 'old news' and to prevent IARC responding as paper was not yet published

Governmental

◆ lobbying governments to oppose restrictions on indoor smoking bans

Source Ong and Glantz 2000

needs champions and charismatic leaders to pool enthusiasm and energy to tackle these issues.

The call for more research should not, however, be seen as arguing for delay in action. There is already an enormous amount known about the health effects of conflict, inequalities, and environmental degradation. Unfortunately, this knowledge is rarely acted upon (Bhutta 2000). Health professionals can do much more as advocates for health, either as individuals or with others, in organizations such as Medact (see www.medact.org, website) (Stott 2001).

Health professionals should thus seek to shape the agenda. We clearly believe that they are stakeholders with a voice that should and can be heard. However we believe that this means avoiding simplistic solutions. Thus the 'public sector good, private sector bad' should be recognized as facile (although we should also strive to convince the many people in the private sector that the converse is equally nonsensical). Similarly, collapsing blame onto a single body, such as the WTO is unlikely to be a constructive way of achieving long-term influence. Instead, we need to draw on the work of those who have explored in detail the complex and changing nature of global inter-relationships (Buse and Walt 2000) as we formulate our own agenda.

This does, however, mean that health professionals must work to get a seat at the table. Too often they engage in endless introspection, preaching to the converted, and remaining outside the corridors of power. Changing this will not be easy, and we will have to earn our place. This means that we must have something positive to contribute to the debate. The challenge is to work with those who do have power to create win–win situations. The opportunities are, however, increasing, as illustrated by the Corporate Initiative for Global Health, organized jointly by the WHO and the World Economic Forum.

Of course there are some powerful interests with whom alliances are impossible, the best example of which is the tobacco industry. There the first challenge is to recognize the nature of the task faced in overcoming the industry's activities. Health professionals everywhere with an interest in tobacco control should take advantage of the release, under court orders, of internal industry documents to discover what the industry has been doing in their country (see www.smoke-screen.org, website). They should also promote and support legal efforts to obtain further disclosure.

Encompassing globalization in public health

Identifying with the opportunities that globalization offers provides a positive start. As outlined above, changing our cognitive view to a one-world paradigm helps in delineation of need, and addressing how the world might seek to reduce the inequities between nations. The global approach to eliminating malaria being promoted by the WHO offers an example. Within countries, a more holistic view is leading to the adoption by development agencies of common funding strategies, termed 'sector wide approaches' (Walt *et al.* 1999).

Dealing with the threats and opportunities associated with globalization is more complicated, and the scope is almost limitless. One approach is to consider issues with a direct influence on health and health services; and other issues with indirect influence on health, such as trade or the environment. This helps in identifying the benefits and harms, the winners and losers, and what can be done to prevent catastrophe or realise benefits.

For many direct influences, identifying the problem is straightforward. For example, infectious diseases spread rapidly, resistance to anti-microbial drugs is a growing problem, and the need for global action is obvious. The opportunities for co-operation seem clear but it is surprising that so little has been done: molecular biology provides a basis for better understanding of the spread of resistance, but this has been little exploited; there is no effective global monitoring of disease outbreaks, and no global standards, methods or strategy for monitoring anti-microbial drug resistance.

For indirect influences, such as the impact of trade on health within nations, the analysis is more complicated. The danger is that we accept bald statements such as 'globalization of trade will exacerbate inequity', or 'the WTO is the new face of imperialism'. We need to consider, at a global level, the positive impacts of these indirect influences, and how these can be maximized; and the potential negative impacts, and how these can be minimized. The problem is that many effects in particular countries cannot be predicted: whilst structural adjustment in Africa was seen initially as the only solution, it was some time before its true effect in worsening poverty and increasing mortality among the poor was recognized. As McMichael points out, health professionals have a role in monitoring the effects of global policies and using this information to advocate change. For example, Wilson and colleagues have examined the impact of the WTO Trade-Related Aspects of Intellectual Property Rights on access to medicine in Thailand, highlighting how this will benefit the USA but restrict access to affordable treatments for HIV in Thailand (Wilson *et al.* 1999). In economic terms, the challenge is to map the externalities: the costs and benefits that accrue to others. Kaul and colleagues describe how such national externality profiles could feed into the global policy agenda (Kaul *et al.* 1999).

Globalization means that we must, as health professionals, view our brief as spanning national boundaries. We need to work with the benefits of globalization, as well as lobbying for change to mitigate against the harmful effects. One part of globalization is localization, bringing back the global lessons to the local context. This means applying them in the situations within which we work. Finally, and most importantly, we need to believe we can make a difference.

References

Abbasi, K. (1999) Free the slaves. *British Medical Journal,* **318,** 1568–9.

Beck, U. (2000) *What is globalization?* Polity, Cambridge.

Bernstein (1996) *Against the gods: the remarkable story of risk.* John Wiley, New York.

Bhutta, Z. A. (2000) Why has so little changed in maternal and child health in South Asia? *British Medical Journal,* **321,** 809–12.

Braverman, H. (1974) *Labor and monopoly capital: the degradation of work in the twentieth century.* Monthly Review Press, New York.

Buse, K. and Walt, G. (2000) Global public–private partnerships: part II – what are the health issues for global governance? *Bulletin WHO,* **78,** 699–709.

Chirimuuta, R. (1989) *AIDS, Africa and racism.* Free Association Books, London.

Cochrane Handbook (2001) in the Cochrane Library, Issue 1, update software, Oxford.

Delamothe, T. and Smith, R. (2001) PubMed Central: creating an Aladdin's cave of ideas. *British Medical Journal,* **322,** 1–2.

Glantz, S., Slade, J., Bero, L. *et al.* (1996) *The cigarette papers.* University of California Press, Berkley.

Jareg, P. and Kaseje, C. O. (1998) Growth of civil society in developing countries: implications for health. *Lancet,* **351,** 819–822.

Kaul, I., Grunberg, I. and Stern, M. A. (1999) *Global public goods, international cooperation in the 21st century,* pp. 450–507. Oxford University Press, Oxford.

Kickbusch, I. and Buse, K. (2001) Global influences and global responses: international health at the turn of the twenty-first century. In *International public health: diseases, programs, systems and policies,* ed. M. H. Myerson, R. E. Black, and A. J. Mills, pp. 667–99. Gaithersburg, Aspen.

Kutumbakam, V. (2000) India's new eight-fold path to the nirvana of globalisation is now unfolding. *India Today,* March 13, 46.

Landes, D. (1998) *The wealth and poverty of nations.* Little, Brown, London.

Lee, K. (1998) Shaping the future of global cooperation: where can we go from here? *Lancet,* **351,** 899–902.

McKee, M. (1999) "Trust me I'm an expert" Why expert advisory committees need to change. *European Journal of Public Health,* **9,** 161–2.

McKee, M., Shkolnikov, V., and Leon, D. A. (2001) Alcohol is implicated in the fluctuations in cardiovascular disease in Russia since the 1980s. *Annals of Epidemiology,* **11,** 1–6.

Ong, E. K. and Glantz, S. A. (2000) Tobacco industry efforts subverting international agency for research on cancer's secondhand smoke study. *Lancet,* **355,** 1253–9.

Pollock, A. M. and Price, D. (2000) Rewriting the regulations: how the World Trade Organisation could accelerate privatisation in health-care systems. *Lancet,* **356,** 1995–2000.

Secretary for State for International Development (1999) Eliminating world poverty: making globalisation work for the poor. White Paper on International Development. HMSO, London.

Sidel, V. W. (1995) The international arms trade and its impact on health. *British Medical Journal,* **311,** 1677–80.

Stiglitz, J. E. (1999) Knowledge as a global public good. In *Global public good: international co-operation in the 21st century,* ed. I. Kaul, I. Grunberg, and M. A. Stern, pp. 308–25. Oxford University Press, New York.

Stott, R. (2001) Global health research. *British Medical Journal,* **322,** 172–3.

Sy, J. H. (1999) Global communications for a more equitable world. In *Global public good: international co-operation in the 21st century,* ed. I. Kaul, I. Grunberg, and M. A. Stern, pp. 326–43. Oxford University Press, New York.

Tweedale, G. (2000) *Magic mineral to killer dust: Turner & Newall and the asbestos hazard.* Oxford University Press, Oxford.

Walt, G. (2001) Global cooperation in international public health. In *International public health: diseases, programs, systems and policies,* ed. M. H. Merson, R. E. Black, and A. J. Mills pp. 667–99. Gaithersburg, Aspen.

Walt, G. (1998) World health: globalisation of international health. *Lancet,* **351,** 434–7.

Walt, G., Pavignani, E., Gilson, L. *et al.* (1999) Managing external resources: are there lessons for SWAPs? *Health Policy and Planning,* **14,** 311–40.

Wilson, D., Cawthorne, P., Ford, N. *et al.* (1999) Global trade and access to medicines: AIDS treatments in Thailand. *Lancet,* **354,** 1893–5.

Wong, J. W. (1998) *Deadly dreams: opium and the arrow war (1856–1860) in China.* Cambridge University Press, Cambridge.

Index

Racketeer Influenced and Corrupt Organization
    Act (USA) 136
radiation and fallout 110–11
railways 7
Reclaim the Streets (direct action group) 8
Red Cross *see* International Committee of the
    Red Cross (ICRC)
refugees 152, 156–9
    see also migration
regulations in health services 31–2
Reinicke, W. H. 24
Report on State of World Food Security (2000)
    100
reporting of communicable disease 51
reproduction 175–6
    family planning actors 180–1
    HIV actors 182–3
    HIV and other sexually transmitted infections
        178–9
    ideological paradigms 183–5
    impact of ideology on reproductive health
        188–90
    International Conference on Population and
        Development 185–8
    international policy actors 179–80
    maternal health actors 181–2
    maternal mortality 177–8
    politics of decisions and ICPD 185–7
    primary health care 183–4
    unwanted pregnancy 176–7
    women's status 184–5
research 22, 26, 32, 44
    biological warfare 115
    by health professionals 204–5
    safe motherhood 182
resistance to antibiotics *see* antibiotics
retail suppliers 97, 99 (**table**)
risks
    collateral health (from climate change) 66
    international transfer of 31, 32–3, 39
    scientific evaluation 72
RJ Reynolds corporation 136
road traffic accidents 87
Rockefeller Foundation 8
Rotblat, Sir Joseph 116
rural and urban living 90–2
Russia 52

SADEC *see* Southern African Development
    Community
Safe Motherhood Conference (Nairobi 1987)
    178, 182
Salm-Net *see* EnterNet
salmonellosis 50, 54
Sanitary and Phytosanitary Standards (SPS)
    101
Saudi Arabia 86
science and arbitration/adjudication on trade
    101–2
Seattle and WTO (1999) 82

security, concept of national 23–4
seed corporations 96 (**table**)
Sen, Amartya 101
Senegal 160–1
shigella 49
shopping patterns 90, 97, 99
Simon, John 75
Singapore 38
SIrUS Project 116–17, 118
slave labour 155–6
slave trade 15, 151
smallpox 2, 15, 115
smoking *see* tobacco
Snow, John 50
society
    and climate change 68
    organization of 14, 16, 70
    see also migration; poverty; shopping
        patterns
soil fertility 61
Solomon Islands 69, 70
Southern African Development Community
    (SADEC) 32
speed of change 5, 14, 18–19, 20, 23
Stanford University Medical Center (USA) 38
Staphylococcus aureus (MRSA) 19
states *see* nation-state concept
statistics, World Health Organization 37
steamship 7
Stiglitz, J. E. 202
stratosphere 66, 67, 73
streptococcus pneumonia 19
stress 19
stroke and mortality 87
sunburn 67
supply chain management 97
surveillance
    international 51–2, 53, 201
    recent developments 55–6
sustainability 64
Sweden 102
Switzerland 36
syphilis 2

TB *see* tuberculosis
Technical Barriers to Trade (TBT) 101
technology
    and carbon dioxide emissions 71
    and information 20, 21, 53, 56
telemedicine 34
telephone communication 5 (**box**)
television 5
territorial transcendence 16–17
Thailand 38, 131 (**box**) 142, 160
thought and globalization 21–3
tobacco 1, 6, 8, 33, 127–8
    advertising 132–3, 132 (**box**) 141–3
    advocacy 141–3
    consultations and conferences 144–5
    countering deception 142 (**box**)